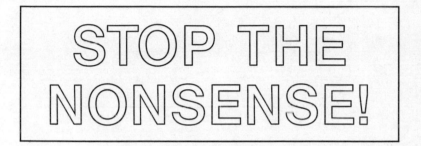

STOP THE NONSENSE!

Health Without Fads

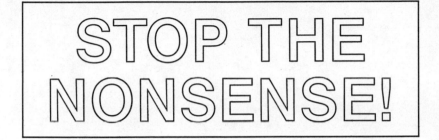

STOP THE NONSENSE!

Health Without Fads

Ezra Sohar, M.D.

SHAPOLSKY PUBLISHERS, INC.
New York

A Shapolsky Book

For any additional information, contact:
Shapolsky Publishers, Inc.
136 West 22nd Street
New York, NY 10011
(212) 633-2022

10 9 8 7 6 5 4 3 2 1

Library of Congress Cataloging-in-Publication Data

Sohar, Ezra, 19–
    Stop the nonsense! : health without fads / Ezra Sohar.
        p.   cm.
    ISBN 1-56171-006-7
    1. Nutrition.   2. Health.   I. Title.
    RA784.S63   1990
    613 — dc20   90-48452

Design and Typography by Smith, Inc., New York

Printed and bound by Graficromo s.a., Cordoba, Spain

Contents

INTRODUCTION

Eternal Life?

Never did so many people live so well as in the affluent western society of the late 20th Century. Never in the past was life so agreeable. People now live longer, food is varied and plentiful, working days are fewer and working hours are shorter. We vacation more and more, traveling in both cars and airplanes, and we take Caribbean and Mediterranean cruises. Television brings the entire world into our homes. Opportunities for self-fulfillment abound. Videocassettes, home computers, and many other amenities make life more meaningful. And, what's more, the agricultural and industrial revolutions of the recent past — and the electronic revolution now evolving before our eyes — are all products of human intelligence and the application of science and technology.

Much has been achieved in this century; many dreams have come true. But we are still far from mankind's fondest dream: eternal life. Well, if not eternal life, most would settle for as long as the Bible says: six-score years. Scientists have already put a man on the moon, so why can't doctors unclog our blood vessels, rid us of arteriosclerosis, and let us live longer? And when so much money has been given for cancer research, why have they still not come up with a cure?

Distrust of Medicine?

Distrust is the gut feeling many people have about medicine. It does not help to point out to them the achievements and successes of medical science in the last century. In every field of medicine these are enormous, by any standard, but they are taken for granted. A well-known plastic surgeon used to say, "Never operate on any patient before taking his picture first." Even people who were severely deformed tend to forget how they looked before the operation. They take their new looks for granted and may even ask you, "What have you actually done for me?" It is possible that doctors, hungry for research grants and funds for better hospitals, have heightened the public's expectations, hinting that solutions for major diseases were just around the corner. So there is today a certain negativism toward doctors and medicine. There may also be other reasons for this credibility gap. Perhaps people feel that doctors charge too much. Some may believe that doctors are more interested in making money than in helping patients. Since less is known about prevention than about healing, doctors are frequently reluctant to give nutritional and life-style advice to healthy people.

Many people have concluded that they are better off fending for themselves. Isn't this the era of self-improvement?

Some approach self-improvement almost hysterically, uncritically applying to themselves whatever nostrum or advice they read or hear about in the media. One day it will be "Coffee causes cancer"—so let's stop drinking coffee. The next day it is: "Meat is unhealthful if cooked at high temperature." So...no more meat for some time. The same goes for eggs, liquid diets, bran, raw vegetables—all have been in and out of vogue. Some people go through all the fads. After spending many hours in the sun to acquire a tan—"to look and feel healthy"—they will then shun the sun completely for fear of skin cancer. Some declare themselves to be born anew, never having felt that well before when they were treated by "conventional" medicine. Some take dangerously exaggerated doses of vitamin C for protection from the common cold, others drink apple vinegar to prevent obesity. Some people will put their faith in holistic medicine or homeopaths, reflexologists, fingernail readers, or other healers. The list is a very long one indeed.

Evaluation of Treatment

"Feeling good" is absolutely no proof of successful therapy. Many people come out of a sauna declaring that they feel refreshed — despite the fact that upon examination every objective indicator will prove the opposite. This point is well illustrated by the experiment related on pages 136–137. In a climatic chamber, temperature and humidity were adjusted to correspond to those in a sauna. This was not told to the experimental subjects, who thought that the purpose of the experiment was to determine "heat load." They did not feel refreshed at all, and complained of discomfort and weakness.

Similarly, it is well known that a doctor's injection of plain water, or even his saying a few compassionate words, will make people "feel much better." This is the power of sugges-tion. All of us are suggestible, and some very much so. In other words, the success or failure of treatment cannot be judged by subjective feelings alone.

The evaluation of drugs or treatments is one of the greatest stumbling blocks in medical research. Even distinguished doc-tors have erred. The following story is attributed to the late Dr. Harvey Cushing, the famous Boston brain surgeon. He once asked an assistant to go over the files of all patients who underwent a certain operation and evaluate its effects. When the young man started reporting his findings, Cushing in-terrupted him and said, "This does not conform with my experience." The young doctor pointed to his figures, insisting: "Dr. Cushing, this *is* your experience."

Several methods have been devised to overcome suggest-

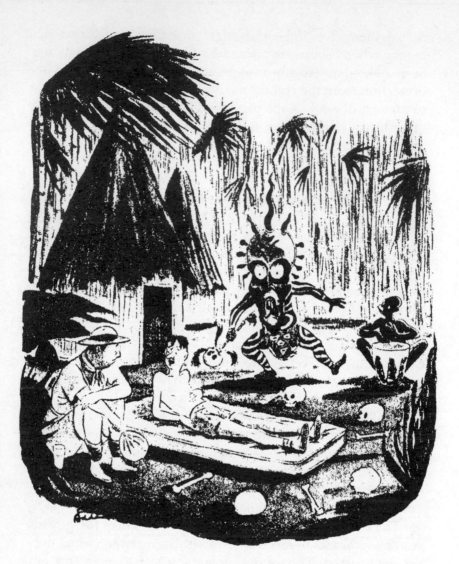

"You won't believe it, but I already feel much better."

(From Charles Addams, *Drawn and Quartered,*
New York: Bantam Books, June 1946)

---

ibility of patients and doctors alike. The so-called "double blind" method is the best known. The pharmacist gives the treating physician identical-looking and -tasting capsules for a group of patients. Only the pharmacist knows which of the patients received a new drug and which a plain powder, or placebo. After a predetermined number of patients have been treated and the results are recorded (who feels better and who doesn't), the code is broken and the treating physician is told who got which compound. The subjective feelings of both doctor or patients are of little meaning, unless they are supported by objective clinical and laboratory findings; that is, unless it is objectively determined that the patients who received the real medicine are those who feel better.

"Conventional" Medicine?

It must immediately be clear that there is no such thing as "conventional medicine," because the term implies that there is also an "unconventional," or "nonconventional," medicine — which does not exist! There is scientific medicine on the one hand and a variety of healers and treatments on the other, the latter of which belong to the realm of superstition.

Once my great-grandfather needed a new suit. The tailor told him how much material to buy, and when he brought the material, the tailor promised a nice three-piece suit. When my great-grandfather came for the first fitting, it was obvious that something had gone wrong. The tailor told him, "Let's sacrifice the vest, and you will have a really good two-piece suit." On the second fitting, things got even worse. After much effort and adjusting, the tailor finally said "We must sacrifice the pants, but I will make you a most beautiful jacket." At this point my great-grandfather said, "It looks as if you don't know how to sew!" And the tailor replied: "That may be, but I still can do it better than you!" Doctors err and make mistakes, but they can still "sew better than you," by providing the only scientifically based medicine available.

Although a considerable body of knowledge concerning illnesses and diseases of the human body has accumulated, there is much doctors still do not yet know. And we must never forget this. As a matter of fact, doctors must tell patients, and the public in general, that we don't know everything!

Nevertheless, medicine is perhaps the only profession in which one must act before all the evidence is in. We cannot tell our patients to come back in ten to twenty years — when more is known about their condition. Nor can we tell them to wait another decade before asking how many eggs they may safely eat. They live now, and we must provide answers now.

What must doctors do when we don't know the full answer? First, we are careful. We do not rush to create a list of do's and don'ts. We explain things clearly and fully, so that patients without basic medical vocabulary will understand what it is on which we base our recommendations. Further, we rely on our experience, remember how many medical beliefs have been discredited in our lifetime. Above all, we must avoid the pitfall of giving "trendy" advice, based uncritically on the most recent findings. Next year, there will be still more recent findings.

This is the spirit in which this book is written. No, there are no sensational breakthroughs to be found in these pages, no fads that will be forgotten before this edition is out of print, no wonder drugs and no list of thirty medications to be taken daily in order to "expand" life.

Rather, this is an account of the state of the art of known, reliable scientific facts. These facts have a bearing on everyday behavior, and may help to prevent disease. Moreover, the facts reported here have one thing in common: They all are accepted in modern medicine.

They are, of course, not all the facts. I have tried to report those that I believe to be relevant. The conclusions are mine, but they correspond, with small variations and nuances, to the prevailing schools of thought accepted by most physicians, though obviously not by all, because different people may arrive at different conclusions from the same or similar sets of facts. I have examined patients in several countries, including Malawi and Uganda in Africa, and New Guinea (Papua) in the Pacific on the one extreme and the United States and Switzerland on the other. For more than three decades I have been treating patients in Israel, patients who come from about, seventy countries, both cold and hot, mountainous and flat, rich and poor. And research done for many years has taught me to evaluate continuing medical discoveries. The recommendations in this book reflect what I have learned from all this experience.

CHAPTER ONE

Preventing Heart Disease

What Is Arteriosclerosis?

Arteriosclerosis is the most widespread disease in Western civilization. It accounts for close to half of human deaths. It is a disease affecting the arteries; i.e., the blood vessels that carry blood from the heart to the periphery (veins carry it back to the heart). Arteriosclerosis causes angina pectoris and heart attacks (myocardial infarction) when the blood vessels supplying the heart muscle are affected, and strokes when the vessels in the brain are diseased. Vessels in other parts of the body are sometimes also affected, but there severe disease is less common.

What actually happens is a narrowing and obstruction of the arteries. It starts with small, yellowish lumps, or plaques, forming on the arteries' inner surface. Early plaque formation was found in autopsies of young American and European soldiers killed in the Korean War—but not found in Asians. It was eventually discovered that very early lesions exist in some teenagers in Western countries. Slowly, the plaques build up, destroying the inner lining of the artery and solidifying by deposits of calcium in the plaques. Finally, the vessel becomes progressively obstructed; its lumen (the passageway of the artery) may even be totally clogged by a blood clot, which forms on the plaque. Clinical manifestations depend on which organ is affected and on the extent of the blocking of the blood vessel.

The disease is almost exclusively limited to areas where European-American civilization prevails. It is seldom found in primitive societies, or in underdeveloped countries in Africa and Asia. One should not forget, of course, that in many of these areas life expectancy is about thirty years, whereas arteriosclerosis usually manifests itself later in life. However, although thirty years is the average, there are old people in these societies, too, and they have little or no arteriosclerosis. On the other hand, immigrants to Western civilization from countries without arteriosclerosis are affected by the disease. This includes blacks, Chinese and Japanese, who came to live in America, in Europe, or in Australia. In a very real sense, it is not a disease of the white man but rather of the white man's civilization.

The Search for Causes

A great deal of statistical, clinical, and experimental medical research has been conducted in the last forty years. The aim is to determine the causes or cause of the disease as a step toward prevention. So far, the results have been partial at best. It is not known why the incidence of heart disease increased to almost epidemic proportions around the 1960s. Nor is it understood why the frequency of heart attacks and stroke declined by some 20 percent or more in the last few years. However, many facts concerning arteriosclerosis *are* known, and will be reported here.

The earliest clues to the causes of arteriosclerosis were

reported after World War II. During the war, in Norway and in other European countries where statistics were available, a steep decrease in heart disease was observed. This occurred in countries where food supply was limited and food stuffs rationed. The high fat content of the arteriosclerotic plaques focused attention on fat in the diet. During the war there was a very significant decrease of fat intake in Norway and other countries where food was scarce. Soon it was discovered that blood cholesterol levels in the general population varied greatly from one country to another. In North America and Western Europe, a level of 180 to 270 milligrams of cholesterol per 100 milliliters of blood was normal, while in African Negroes, living on their traditional diets, the average blood cholesterol level was about 120 to 140 mg per 100 ml blood. One could almost tell the relative standard of living of any country by the average blood cholesterol level of its inhabitants.

In 1948, a well-planned prospective study began among the inhabitants of Framingham, Mass., and is being followed up to the present. The researchers of this study examine prospectively, every two years, the residents of Framingham from every possible aspect and angle, in relation to heart disease. This is, without doubt, the most extensive, long-lasting and best-conceived epidemiological study ever undertaken in an attempt to determine the influence of various risk factors, including external factors, on the development of heart disease. This study established that the higher the blood cholesterol level, the greater was the likelihood of having a heart attack. Many years later, it has been concluded, from the findings of a large-scale experiment conducted simultaneously in several cities in the United States, that a reduction in blood cholesterol levels decreases the incidence of heart attacks.

Some people with high blood cholesterol grow old without ever experiencing a heart attack, while others, whose cholesterol level is normal or even low, may suffer one or have a stroke. Many other factors were investigated and the conclusion was reached that arteriosclerosis was a disease with many contributing causes. These are called "risk factors." The following risk factors are known: smoking; obesity; high blood cholesterol; hypertension; diabetes; heredity; male sex. The term "risk factor" does not imply that a person having any of them will automatically, sooner or later, have a heart attack. It means, however, that he or she is at greater risk than someone without the risk factor.

Smoking

There is no doubt, today, that heavy cigarette smoking is the number-one risk factor, capable of precipitating heart attacks in people who have no other risk factors. Heart attacks have been reported in heavy smokers between the ages twenty and thirty, a rarity among nonsmokers. Smoking one pack of cigarettes daily for a prolonged period of time shortens life expectancy by an average of about four years; two packs a day will shorten it by approximately seven years. Smoking is discussed more extensively in Chapter Seven.

Obesity

Obesity (having excessive fat tissue) does not directly increase the risk of heart attacks but, predisposes a person to cardio-vascular disease, mainly by raising fat levels in the blood and by causing hypertension. In this way it promotes the development of arteriosclerosis. The risk of obesity is directly related to the degree of overweight, starting at about 20 percent above the normal mean weight. Obesity is discussed in detail in Chapter Eight.

Hypertension and Diabetes

Hypertension, or high blood pressure, as well as diabetes can not now be prevented, but their harmful effects can be reduced by proper care and treatment. If there is any merit in yearly medical checkups, it is to a large extent in early diagnosis of these two serious diseases. Consistent treatment of hypertension can usually keep blood pressure close to normal levels. In most cases of diabetes, blood sugar can be controlled by the patient's own constant monitoring under his physician's supervision. By such care the risk of heart attacks can be decreased.

Heredity

While our efforts can have an effect on the above-mentioned risk factors, it appears that there is not very much we can do about heredity. In some cases there is a family history of heart attacks and no other known risk factor is present. In most cases this is not so: People with a family history of heart disease should be thoroughly examined early in life, and one or more of the known risk factors will probably be found. Appropriate treatment will then minimize or postpone the risk for many years.

Sex

Myocardial infarction is considerably more common in males and occurs, very often, at a younger age than in females. It seems that female sex hormones have, in some as yet undetermined way, a protective influence on the coronary arteries. After menopause (arrest of regles) the incidence of myocardial infarction in women increases steeply.

Cumulative Effect of Risk Factors

Each risk factor increases the chances of having a heart attack by a certain percentage. In people having two or more risk factors, the chances of having a myocardial infarction or a cerebral hemorrhage or thrombosis, are cumulative, meaning that they are the sum total of the effect of each of the risk factors present. It follows that people having two or more risk factors, must make efforts to reduce those of the risk factors, which can be reduced by diet, behavior, or medical treatment.

What Determines Blood Cholesterol Level

Of all the factors involved in the development of arteriosclerosis and heart attacks, most attention by far has been focused on cholesterol. Extensive research has been conducted on cholesterol and other fatty materials in the blood, trying to identify and trace the danger and find ways to neutralize it.

Despite forty years of intensive and widespread research, and hundreds of millions of dollars, much remains unclear. There is still controversy as to the precise role played by cholesterol in the development of arteriosclerosis, its relative importance, and the ways of reducing its level in the blood.

Cholesterol is not a fat but a fat-like substance. Usually ingested together with animal fats, mostly saturated, it is dissolved by fat solvents. The blood level of cholesterol is *not* determined by the amount of cholesterol eaten—certainly not exclusively so. The most important determinant is heredity. Some people have a higher blood cholesterol level than others, even if they eat exactly the same diet as their friends; this is due to genetically transmitted disorders.

Much of the cholesterol in food is destroyed during digestion. Our own blood cholesterol is formed in the liver. The amount produced depends more upon the content of *saturated fat* (see page 56) in our diet than on its cholesterol content. Cholesterol is usually excreted in the bile. In the excretion process there may also be individual differences that have an impact on the blood cholesterol level. By adhering religiously to a diet completely devoid of saturated fat and of cholesterol, blood levels can be reduced at most by some 25 percent.

Dieting a Limited Success

Diets low in saturated fat and low in cholesterol have been recommended for decades. Their success has not been very impressive, for several reasons. First and foremost, for people living in an affluent society, where food supply is abundant, it is extremely difficult to adhere to a diet, day in and day out. Saturated fat is found in many of the foods we are accustomed to eating and fond of eating. One can abstain for a limited period of time—but forever?

Another drawback is the general public's lack of knowledge. People don't always know what a cooked dish contains, nor are they certain whether the fat in various foods is "saturated" or not. In many cases, people follow a "condensed" procedure, giving up eating eggs and red meat—believing that this is all they have to change in their diet to enhance their health and promote longevity.

Furthermore, traditional eating habits are hard to change. It is very difficult, almost impossible, to bring about radical changes in the eating habits of whole populations. It is remarkable how people adhere to culinary traditions. A good case in point are the Italians who immigrated to the United States. Their children and grandchildren still cherish Italian cuisine. New food items are being added only slowly. The same phenomenon has been observed with other immigrants to America and elsewhere.

If so, how come that the incidence of arteriosclerotic heart disease is higher in various immigrant groups in the U.S.A., than it was in their native countries? This can best be explained by citing the Bedouins (nomads of the deserts of the Middle East) as an example. The Bedouins are sheep and goat herding desert dwellers. However, their food consists mainly of pita (a flat home-baked bread), legumes, onions, oil, etc. They like sheep and goat meat very much, but in their natural state they could not afford to eat meat more than a very few times yearly. Naturally, the level of their blood cholesterol was very low. Once they come to live in better economic circumstances, they stick to what they like and are used to, but now they eat meat with a high fat content, prepared in the same way it was done in the desert, three times weekly or even every day, instead of four or five times a year. They are still eating their favorite food—but now it is much richer in saturated fat. The same holds true for Italian immigrants to America. They still like pasta, but now more of all the expensive ingredients is added: cheese, meat, and butter—all very high in saturated fat.

In an attempt to decrease the incidence of arteriosclerosis and the resulting heart attacks, it has been suggested that the whole nation should greatly curtail the intake of foods containing saturated fats. To propose a drastic change in eating habits to whole nations, it must be unequivocally established that a change in diet is absolutely essential and that no damage to health will occur in some other systems or organs of the body. The recommendations must be clear qualitatively and quantitatively, and compliance must be feasible. Physicians and scientists have reservations concerning the first two points, and in practice the problem of compliance proves much more difficult than expected.

Let us consider the example of tooth hygiene. Dentists and health workers have told us for several decades that sweets cause tooth decay. The damaging influence of sweets has been definitely proven. Furthermore, the entire population has been made aware of it and is convinced that this is true. Nevertheless, consumption of sweets does not show signs of decreasing. I suspect that even some dentists, going to visit their young nieces or nephews, will bring them chocolate and other candy. It is not that people do not want their children to have healthy teeth, but they are not willing to pay the price of giving up sweets for good.

Presumably, people are more ready to sacrifice parts of their diet to prevent heart attacks, but at what age? It is true that, after a heart attack, elderly people will usually be willing to follow almost any diet their doctors prescribe. But what about teenagers, or people feeling well and in the prime of life? If a diet reducing blood cholesterol is to be effective, it must be started very early in life—not after arteriosclerosis has long played havoc with the heart.

The majority of citizens will not heed advice that calls for drastic changes in general eating habits. Physicians should take this into account, and their recommendations should be those that can be followed. Otherwise, people will pay lip service but try to forget about the whole thing during mealtime.

There seems to be no obvious risk involved in increasing the unsaturated fat content in our diet; some societies consume unsaturated fat almost exclusively. However, their total fat intake is much lower than ours. If the fat consumption of Western societies were reduced from the present 100 to 120 grams daily to about 80 grams—and half of it unsaturated—we would be perfectly safe, according to all the available evidence. On the other hand, it is questionable whether it would be wise to eliminate saturated fat entirely, even if it were feasible. About 30 to 40 grams of saturated fat per day is not harmful. By eating that much, we do not run the risk of lacking some as yet unidentified food ingredient our body may need.

Must Everybody Diet?

The major question, of course, is the efficacy of a drastic change in diet. Is it essential and is it a must for everyone? Proponents of a radical change of diet, claim that this will reduce the number of heart attacks by 50 percent. However, the incidence of heart attacks, after having risen for several decades, began to decrease in the late 1970s. Now it is about 20 percent less than it was at its peak during the 1960s and is still declining. It is not known what brought about this happy development, but it can hardly be attributed to dietary changes, which, according to statistics, are negligible. The most likely explanation is a decrease in cigarette smoking and, perhaps also, modern treatment of hypertension, although available data do not support the latter. Medical history knows other instances when incidence of disease increased or decreased without any obvious explanation. Gout, for instance, was much more prevalent at the beginning of the century. The drastic decrease in incidence of cancer of the uterine cervix is also not fully accounted for.

Evidence from the Framingham study (see page 11), shows clearly that the incidence of heart attacks rises progressively when blood cholesterol levels exceed 220 to 240 mg. per 100 ml. It follows that those whose blood cholesterol level is below 220 mg. are not required to change their diet drastically. Only about 20 percent of the population have blood cholesterol levels above 240 mg. As was already mentioned, a strict diet alone can bring it down by a maximum of 25 percent. It follows that a cholesterol-reducing diet must be observed more conscientiously the higher the blood cholesterol level, and that it is advisable to check blood cholesterol level every two years or so.

Eggs

Eggs are of a high cholesterol content and therefore a favorite target of attack by dietary reformers. However, no close correlation between egg consumption and blood cholesterol levels has been found. In the Framingham study, for instance, people were divided into groups according to whether they ate half an egg, one egg, or up to two and a half eggs daily. No correlation was found between the number of eggs consumed and blood levels of cholesterol—nor with the incidence of coronary heart disease. It seems that there is no reason to shun eggs specifically for their cholesterol content. Nevertheless, each egg also contains approximately 6 to 7 grams of saturated fat, depending on its size (7 grams are about a 1/4 of an ounce). For *this* reason, eating too many eggs is not desirable. One of my patients, a chicken farmer, ate 15 to 20 eggs daily. He had a heart attack while in his early thirties.

Studies on the direct influence of red meat on heart attacks are lacking. It appears that it has been specifically denounced because of its relatively high cholesterol content. But interpretation of present knowledge indicates that eggs and all meats are better evaluated according to their saturated-fat content.

A Reasonable Diet—
An Attainable Goal

In Western Europe and North America, daily fat consumption is about 100 to 120 gr. (3 1/2 to 4 oz.) per person. Except in Italy and Spain, more than two-thirds of the dietary fat is saturated. The sources of saturated fat are as follows: milk and dairy products such as butter, cheese, cream, etc.; beef, pork, lamb, and poultry; eggs; peanuts; most margarines; cocoa fat and cocoa butter; and of course all the products containing these ingredients, such as chocolate, pastries, cakes, ice cream (except sherbets), many kinds of sweets, etc. (See table on pages 57–58.)

It is unthinkable to ask whole populations to deprive themselves completely of these foods. It would be an unattainable goal, and also unnecessary. Just the same, there is value in cutting daily fat intake to about 80 grams (2 2/3 oz.), *not more than* half of it saturated. This could be achieved without too great a sacrifice in the taste of food and without major changes in eating habits. Here are some suggestions:

(1) Drink milk of 1 percent fat content instead of regular milk, which contains 3 to 4 percent. You "save" between 20 to 30 gr. (2/3 to 1 oz.) on every quart.

(2) Don't use butter or margarine for frying and cooking, but instead use one of the unsaturated oils, like soybean, cottonseed, sunflower, sesame, olive, or corn oil. Sandwiches can be spread with mayonnaise or mustard instead of butter or margarine *(mayonnaise, prepared with one egg for one cup of oil, is almost entirely unsaturated)*.

(3) For frying, use Teflon-coated pans. You need only a fraction of the oil that is necessary for frying in a regular pan.

(4) Buy lean meat and, when preparing it, trim off any visiable fat. Remove the skin of chicken: It contains a large part of the fat. Broiling and barbecuing are preferred methods of preparing meat, since they remove some of the fat.

(5) Instead of peanuts, serve almonds and other nuts.

(6) Instead of chocolate, eat sweets with less fat, such as hard candy, halva, jelly beans, etc., and dried fruit. Instead of regular ice cream, try sherbet or tofutti.

(7) Cake recipes that do not contain much fat are preferable.

(8) When preparing your own salad dressing, use no other fat but oil.

(9) Fish contains less fat than meat, and the fat in most fish —seafish—is unsaturated. Several times weekly, serve fish instead of meat.

Adhering to these recommendations will reduce fat intake, especially saturated-fat intake, without requiring too drastic a change in the habitual diet.

Legumes to Reduce
High Cholesterol

Recent studies in many parts of the world have indicated that dietary plant fibers from cereals, vegetables, and legumes lower blood cholesterol. When food with high fiber content was given experimentally over several months to a group of people with high blood cholesterol, a significant reduction in blood cholesterol occurred.

It appears that legumes (beans, chick peas, lentils, etc.) are more effective than cereals and vegetables. It is not clear whether this property of legumes is due to their fiber content only, or whether some other substances, specific to the legume family, play a role. But it seems advisable for people with a high blood cholesterol to include in their daily diet at least 50 gr. of dry beans or chick peas. This can be safely recommended, because it cannot be harmful. In addition, other high fiber foods should be included in the diet.

If the reports on the blood cholesterol-lowering effect of legumes are corroborated in large-scale tests, this may well become the preferential dietary method of control for those whose blood cholesterol level is above 220 mg. It might even allow them to eliminate fewer of their favorite saturated fat-containing foods.

Physical Activity and
Arteriosclerosis

Many scientists and physicians believe that a lack of physical activity is one of the factors that enhances arteriosclerosis. In modern urban life, especially in Europe and America, there is much less physical activity than in the world's more primitive societies. In the latter societies arteriosclerosis is virtually non-existent. It therefore appears that in some way physical activity prevents, or delays, arteriosclerosis.

While a certain amount of muscular activity is beneficial to the proper functioning of the body, there is little hard evidence of a direct effect of physical activity on arterio-sclerosis (see more extensive discussion on pages 26–27 and 31–32). There are indications that physically active people may survive a heart attack better than others; they also have a higher threshold of anginal pain (namely, physically active persons, in whom narrowing of the arteries supplying blood to the heart develops, are capable of a higher level of physical effort before pain starts). But it has not been proven that jogging or other athletic activity can arrest arteriosclerosis. Signs and symptoms of arteriosclerosis have been found even in many marathon runners.

CHAPTER TWO

How Much Exercise?

Heredity and Environment

Much of the size, look, and functions of our body are genetically determined, although genetic determination is not absolute. External factors have their influence. An example is the onset of sexual maturity in women, as manifested by the menarche, the first menstruation. In affluent societies it occurs in most women between the ages of 12 and 13. But at the beginning of this century, mean age at first menstruation in England, Sweden, and other European countries was 15 or even 16 years—as it still is in some underdeveloped countries. We now know that for female sexual maturation to occur at the genetically predetermined age, 12 to 13, the girls' nutritional status must be good. In other words, undernourishment postpones menarche for years.

The same is true of height. It was a common observation

that children of immigrants from Europe to the United States or Australia grew to be significantly taller than their parents. Many of their parents lacked vitamins and possibly other nutrients in their growing years, and therefore did not attain their genetically determined height. This phenomenon was very pronounced in Japan after 1950. The living standard rose and nutrition improved. The younger generation today is, on the average, 6 to 7 inches taller than the previous one.

Well-fed and well-cared-for young people will usually stop growing sometime between the ages of 16 and 21. The height they will have reached is final, and there is no way to add to it or reduce it. The same goes for intelligence. People can learn to use their brain, they can acquire knowledge and techniques; but intelligence itself cannot be improved on, or at best very little. This holds true for nearly all other systems of the body.

Muscles — Tissue in Constant Flux

The only exception to this general rule is muscular tissue. It is of course also genetically determined, but the individual's maximum limit is rarely achieved, even by athletes. While in other systems of the body the development achieved by interaction of genetic and external factors is final, *muscular tissue is in constant flux.* Muscles develop when used and atrophy when not used. Their size and ability and upper limit of function depend on the performance required of them. The female uterus is a very good example. It is composed almost exclusively of muscles. Its normal weight is about 50 grams, but during pregnancy it grows to surprising proportions, reaching the weight of 1 kilogram; i.e., 20 times its pre-pregnancy weight! After a mother gives birth, the uterus contracts and after a few months reverts to its previous weight.

Or take the case of an athlete whose leg muscles are developed to a remarkable degree. If he fractures his leg, it is immobilized with a cast. When the cast is removed, complete immobilization has shrunk the muscles to a poor, even grotesque, semblance of their former state. This clearly shows that muscles are functional tissue. Muscle development is enhanced by male sex hormones. Although women athletes have achieved remarkable ability, sheer muscular power remains the only realm in which men have clear superiority over women. With age, diminishing blood supply, and disuse, muscles begin to shrink gradually, producing some of the changes in body appearance that are typical of old age.

Muscles are underdeveloped in people with a sedentary way of life, and can be overdeveloped in weightlifters and others. Furthermore, muscles do not develop to the same degree throughout the body. When athletes train, all their muscles grow but some grow more than others. It depends on the type of training. The muscle groups used for swimming, running, football, or boxing are not the same. A trainer can tell by the appearance of his muscles what an athlete has trained for.

The effect of training is not restricted to muscles; the heart and lungs are also involved. During exercise the number of respirations per minute increases, and with it the depths of respiration, meaning the amount of air exchanged with each respiration. In this way the amount of oxygen introduced into the blood is greatly increased. The heart muscle too grows with exercise, and is trained to be able, when needed, to pump more blood per unit of time into the circulatory system, supplying the muscles with all the oxygen needed to perform the additional work load. The output of the whole system can be measured and is expressed as VO2 max., the maximal capacity of the body to utilize oxygen in a unit of time, indicating the maximal amount of energy the body can produce in a unit of time. This capacity may be twice as great in exercisers as in sedentary people. This measurement is the best quantitative expression of *physical fitness.*

The Rewards of Exercise

Athletic activity is rewarded by physical fitness, accompanied by a feeling of well-being. In primitive societies, physical fitness was held in much higher esteem than in our society. It was essential for survival in war, in hunting, and in food gathering. Up until the beginning of this century, most people needed physical fitness for earning their living. Gradually, however, muscle power was replaced by machines. Today the number of people engaged in physically exerting work decreases steadily, and, for most of those who are still working physically, the nature of that work is less demanding.

Though one could go through life in modern society almost without moving a muscle, this would hardly be an enjoyable life. A certain degree of muscular development is necessary for a good posture and a nice figure. And what about the many athletic pleasures of life—such as dancing, surfing, cycling, mountain climbing, hiking with a backpack, and so forth? Even to catch a subway when in a hurry or to walk up a staircase without panting one needs physical fitness. Enjoyable sexual activity requires also a certain degree of strength. And of course there is the pleasure of sport as such. It constitutes an important and pleasurable part of young peoples' lives. Children are spontaneously attracted to outdoor games. Youngsters fill the playgrounds in schools and neighborhoods.

Clearly, exercise betters the quality of life.

Exercise and Health

The connection between exercise and health depends upon our definition of health. If we take health to denote a full life, enjoying all capacities, physical and intellectual, then the answer is clearly pro-exercise. However, if the question is whether sport helps prevent disease or promote longevity, the answer becomes much more complicated.

It stands to reason that a certain amount of muscular activity has a beneficial influence on the body's functions. Circulation is enhanced; the heart-lung mechanism is kept fit; a larger percentage of what we eat is "burned" as fuel and not stored as fat. There may also be a long-term stabilizing influence on the appetite and better sleep induced by physical tiredness. Physical fitness also diminishes the risk of accidents. An agile person has a supple body and a better chance of escaping from an onrushing car, falling without injury, or regaining balance when slipping, etc. Beyond this, clear-cut evidence that exercise promotes health is scarce. It does not help to prevent cancer or infectious diseases. It is too early to evaluate whether there is any effect of exercise on the immune system.

It should also be kept in mind that active sports produce a remarkable number of accidents, usually affecting the muscle and bones. In a study reported in the *Journal of the American Medical Association* in 1979, it is estimated that football alone may produce more than one million injuries per year in the U.S.A. To be sure, most of them are trivial and heal completely, but among the million there must be several thousand injuries that are of a more serious nature. Permanent injuries, or damage to bones, joints, spine, and other organs cannot be discounted. The amount of serious damage differs among the various sports, and in some, such as boxing, it may be quite high.

Exercise and Heart Disease

The major question — not devoid of controversy — is the effect of exercise on heart disease, especially in the prevention or slowing of development of arteriosclerosis, thus promoting longevity. One much-cited study, begun in the 1950s and conducted for 22 years on 6,000 longshoremen in the San Francisco Bay area, showed that those engaged in strenuous, very vigorous work had significantly fewer heart attacks than those engaged in medium or light work. This study, and some other investigations on a smaller scale, was a keystone for physicians in advising everyone to continue vigorous physical activity beyond middle and into old age. However, since vigorous physical *work* is virtually nonexistent, the advice really refers to exercise and sports. And the protective effect of vigorous physical activity lasts only as long as it is exercised and disappears shortly after it is stopped. This is well documented by follow-up studies of professional athletes, champions, etc. As a group, they do not have a smaller incidence of arteriosclerotic heart disease, and do not live longer than the population at large.

Why do people stop vigorous exercise at a certain point? Many probably do so because it becomes too hard for them — in other words, because of the development of arteriosclerosis, in spite of the exercise. It has been proven that some marathon runners and others engage in strenuous exercise, but nevertheless develop arteriosclerosis and heart attacks. Jogging and even marathon running does not assure protection. There is growing concern about the incidence of what is termed sudden death during or very shortly after exercise. This may occur in any age group. In many cases of young people, death was traced to a hidden unsymptomatic heart disease. But the question remains whether they would have died had they not exercised vigorously. In middle-aged and older people, sudden death was almost always traced to arteriosclerotic heart disease. It is the consensus of opinion that exercise increases greatly the risk of sudden death in subjects with heart disease. People believing that exercise will decrease their chances of having a heart attack have swelled the ranks of joggers, squash players, and other sportsmen.

When does a person start thinking about heart attacks? In high school and college, students have different things to think about. Then in middle age, when the first symptoms of arteriosclerosis occur, such as chest pain, people become alarmed and start to exercise. This is dangerous. Here are people who have not exercised since they left college; their coronary arteries are not what they used to be. Suddenly launching into a demanding training program may achieve the exact opposite of what was intended. It is advisable to be medically examined before beginning to exercise after a nonphysical interval of several years. But even a thorough medical examination, including an ECG (electrocardiogram) done during physical effort, will not always detect coronary narrowing. Any training program should therefore be started *slowly and gradually*.

Jogging

Mass participation in jogging is relatively recent. It is fashionable and has a reputation of being "good for your heart." Young and old are puffing along the road, many of them with visible effort. But there is very little evidence that jogging decreases hypertension or the incidence of heart attacks. On the other hand, there is a growing list of adverse consequences. Sudden deaths from heart attacks occur. The chances of having a heart attack while jogging are about five times greater than when one is at rest. It has even happened that joggers became victims of car accidents, since people engaged in strenuous physical effort may not be sufficiently alert to their surroundings. Injuries to ankles, knees, and spine occur — some of them leaving permanent damage. Many other pathological conditions, specific to jogging, even a temporary kidney disease, have been identified.

Taking all these factors into consideration, it is questionable whether any possible advantages of jogging outweigh the disadvantages. It seems that the human body was not designed to run long distances. When we are walking, one foot is always on the ground, whereas when we are running both feet are in the air for a certain length of time at each step. This is the main difference between walking and running. When we walk, we put the stepping foot down, and the body's weight is still supported by the other foot. The weight is shifted onto the forward foot slowly, without jolting. Conversely, when running, the whole body's weight rests on one foot, which comes stamping down on the ground with each step. This takes its toll on the ligaments and joints of the legs and of the spine. Apparently they were not designed for such harsh treatment.

There is another disadvantage to jogging. Despite its present popularity, it is obviously not suitable for everyone. Very few people can keep it up for years, and certainly not for decades. Only a very limited number of middle-aged people continue jogging, even if they did jog before. It is not the kind of exercise that becomes part of a way of life and that can be safely recommended to all.

Walking

Walking can increase one's physical fitness almost to the same degree as running, without the dangers and discomforts inherent in running. The walking pace can be adjusted individually. Once it is acquired as a life habit, anyone can continue walking, even into old age. Throughout his long life, President Harry S. Truman used to take brisk walks—which kept the White House reporters at his side short of breath.

By "walking" I do not mean a slow stroll or a leisurely "constitutional" with the dog on the leash. In an experimental walking program, which I published together with my research associates in 1980, while jogging was at its height, in the *Journal of the American Medical Association,* we reported that people's physical fitness rose significantly within a short period of time when the participants were asked to walk for 30 minutes, five times a week, at a pace of 3 miles per hour; that is, they walked 1.5 miles each time. During the walk they carried a six-pound load. Average physical fitness of the participants increased by about 20 percent. In those who continued the walking for another few weeks, with an increased load of twelve pounds, physical fitness continued to rise.

Walking has great advantages. It is not dangerous. The initial effort is relatively small, unlike that of jogging, squash, and other forms of exercise that have a high threshold of effort (even beginners immediately have to exercise strenuously). Even tennis, if started in middle age, may be too exacting, as it requires short, concentrated bursts of great effort. Furthermore, one can walk nearly everywhere and at all times. No special paraphernalia or roads are necessary. It can easily become a way of life, and it does nor need to disrupt other everyday routines. Though it seems reasonable to take a walk in the evening, it can also be done in the morning, on the way to or from work, while carrying groceries home from shopping—at many convenient times and places. It is not advisable, however, to take a brisk walk after a meal.

People who take up walking will often walk for more than

their daily planned exercise. When people become used to walking, they will think nothing of walking half a mile or more to the store or post office, leaving the car at home.

Exercise and Advanced Age

With advance in age, a decrease in functional capacity occurs. Every year, after reaching adulthood, the heart's capacity as the body's blood pump decreases by 1 percent. Blood vessels become narrower and less flexible. The velocity of the blood in the blood vessels at age 60 is decreased by a third. The amount of air that the lungs are capable of inhaling in a unit of time decreases to about half at age 75. And, perhaps surprising, after the age of 30 the number of muscle fibers decreases by some 3 to 5 percent every decade. Decrease of calcium in the bones occurs, too, with age.

There is, so far, no means to arrest or reverse these processes. *This is the way of all flesh.* But physical activity can slow them, and even develop compensation mechanisms. In fact, the *only* way is physical activity — but it must be adjusted to age.

People above 60 should never embark on any physical activity program except gradually and after medical examination. It is advisable to examine one's pulse rate during exercise, to make sure that the heart is not overloaded. Never exceed 60 to 70 percent of the maximal allowed pulse rate for each age. Deduct your age from the figure 220 and figure out the percentage. Example for age 70: 220 – 70 = 150. Sixty percent of 150 is 90, 70 percent is 105. It follows that the pulse rate during exercise should not exceed, in this example, 90 to 105.

Walking and Swimming

Suggested types of activity: Walking for half an hour at a rate of 3 miles an hour, four to five times weekly, is appropriate for elderly people. If your pulse rate does not reach 60 percent of the maximal allowed rate, the speed of walking can be increased. Another advisable activity is swimming for half an hour instead of walking. The pulse rate during swimming should not exceed 60 percent of that allowed.

Gymnastics

Furthermore, it is advisable to do gymnastics for several minutes each day, irrespective of what method is used. The aim is to prevent "rusting" of the joints. All joints, from the neck down, should be successively activated. Again, start gradually and don't exert yourself too much.

Bending, with Weight

If time is available and the will is there, you may want to try to strengthen your muscles. Put a small sack of sand, weighing two pounds, on the back of the foot (while sitting), and straighten the knee, repeating the action for several minutes. Gradually the weight can be increased to several pounds. This strengthens the quadriceps muscle, located on the anterior side of the upper leg. There are also exercises for the arms. But do not overdo it, for it may be dangerous.

Physical activity is very important in advanced years, but it must be practiced sensibly, and not in competition with the young! It will give you not the "spring of youth," but perhaps pleasure and a better quality of life.

Summary

Our affluent, technological society has brought about changes in our lives that have a direct influence on our bodies. While many of these changes can be regarded as positive from the physiological point of view, some of them are negative. In modern society, the locomotor system (the system responsible for the body's movements—primarily muscles and bones) is underutilized, with the consequence that physical fitness is low. There is no doubt that physical fitness is an integral part of a full and enjoyable life. Exercise is the only reasonable way to acquire physical fitness, since in our society mechanical power has replaced muscular energy.

Though it seems reasonable to assume that physical fitness

promotes good health, there is little hard-core evidence that it can prevent diseases or prolong life. Some studies have shown that very vigorous physical exertion decreases the number of heart attacks. Beyond a certain age, however, vigorous exercise carries with it many dangers, including sudden death from heart disease. There is also evidence that jogging and marathon running are responsible for a long list of injuries and do not ensure immunity from arteriosclerosis. Starting on a vigorous training program in middle age, after having experienced some chest pain or other symptoms of heart disease, is downright dangerous.

Under these circumstances, the most logical advice would be that children and young people should engage in the sports or exercise of their choice. They should also be protected from injuries and dangers by medical examinations, protective gear, and wise supervision. As one's years advance, one should keep up a way of life that maintains physical fitness with minimum danger. Regular walking seems a reasonable way of achieving this goal.

CHAPTER THREE

Good Stress, Bad Stress

Is Stress a By-Product of Modern Life?

Stress has by now become a household word. Many of our troubles and problems, including quite a number of diseases, are often being blamed on "the stress of modern life." These are the so-called diseases of civilization, and they include ulcers, high blood pressure, arteriosclerosis, and diabetes. It is generally lamented that stress is the villain of modern life, the price we pay for the comfort and advantages of our civilization.

In a book published in London a few years ago, advising the public on how to maintain good health, we find the following sentences: "A competitive modern businessman is in a worse situation, from the point of view of stress, than a primitive hunter whose prey has run away. . . . It seems that the social stress situations without outlet occurred only very rarely in the ancient primitive society." The assumption that stress is much more common in modern society than it was in ancient times is widely shared. But this has in no way been proven and, of course, the question remains: When did "modern times" begin?

A distinguished British physician wrote, more than a hundred years ago, of a disease whose cause was unknown at the time: "This disease is one of the penalties we pay for out boasted progress. There is reason to believe that . . . modern modes of life have something to do with its propagation. . . . The struggle for existence has become a melee. . . ." Years later, the disease he referred to was found to be due to an infection and had nothing whatsoever to do with the "struggle for existence"; it was is in no way connected with business.

The words of a Chinese philosopher, some 4600 years ago, are even more poignant: "But the present world is a different one. Griefs, calamity, and evil cause inner bitterness. . . . Evil influences strike from early morning until late at night . . . they injure the mind and reduce its intelligence, and they also injure the muscle and the flesh."

It seems that "modern times" have been with us for at least the last several thousand years. Nevertheless, each generation seems to believe that it is the first, or at most the second, to suffer from the "terrible stress of our times."

Life in Primitive Societies

These claims cannot be substantiated when one gets acquainted with accounts of real life in primitive societies. There are many authentic reports of life as it was in the Stone Age. This can be inferred from what has been observed in New Guinea and some nonliterate societies in Africa, Asia, and South America.

A unique document has recently been published by an Italian anthropologist. It is the story of an eleven-year-old girl, kidnapped by primitive tribes in the jungles of the Amazon. She succeeded in escaping after 20 years. It is a firsthand, tape-recorded account of the life she led among the savages. Her account tells that these people have virtually no possessions (except their bows and hammocks), depend almost exclusively on hunting for survival, are exposed to wild animals, haunted by superstitions, and are in constant, unrelenting tribal warfare. Women cry for a good part of their lives, out of frustration and unresolved social-stress situations, involving either themselves or their families.

The notion that primitive societies live in harmony and pastoral calm has absolutely no support in reality, and is totally opposed to what knowledge has been accumulated about life in such societies. It is likely that even the most competitive and ambitious man today is exposed to considerably fewer stress situations and, within these situations, to a lesser degree of stress.

Physiology of General Stress

Stress gives rise to well-defined physiological manifestations. Blood pressure rises, pulse rate quickens, blood clots more easily, certain white blood cells decrease in number, and so forth. This is the body's reaction to *every kind of stress,* physical or mental. Be it an athlete about to compete, a student taking an examination, or an actor about to go on the stage, the physiological reaction is basically the same.

But although the physiological reaction to every kind of stress is the same, the outcome differs. A soldier will not die of fright during an enemy assault, but he may have a heart attack when he is unexpectedly informed of the death of a close relative. Or take politicians in high office. They have tremendous responsibility in national crises, in peace, and in war. They get little sleep and put in many hours of work; they confront emergencies; and they do *not* generally succumb to stress. Apparently, as long as they are in power, all these things do not harm them—on the contrary they seem to thrive on them. Without stress reaction, which mobilizes the physical reserves of the body, no athlete and no actor would be able to give his or her best performance. These are situations in which stress reaction is not only harmless but is clearly of positive value, essential for survival and achievement.

It is relevant here to cite a leading article published in the prestigious British medical journal *The Lancet,* in March 1983. The paper deals with a possible causative relation between stress and hypertension: "In general, researchers have been resistant to become involved in discussions of stress, mainly because there is no accepted standard for measuring it. Furthermore, many enthusiasts for the stress hypothesis are, to put it mildly, unscientific."

Stress cannot be quantitatively measured, nor can one's reaction to it. It seems to affect different persons differently. Some will have a stress reaction to a very mild stimulus, others will experience it only when the stimulus is very strong. Stress is not a rare occurrence. It affects all of us, very frequently, from the very moment of birth, which is in itself a very severe stress on the fetus. From then on we experience stress throughout life: in school, later on the job, in our family life, in rearing children, and in many daily-recurring, other situations like reading a newspaper, watching television, etc., etc. Under these circumstances it is easy to blame every disease whose causative factors have not yet been completely elucidated or every discomfort or headache on stress—even though there is very little evidence to support these claims.

To Die of Grief

In the Bible, Jacob is quoted as having said to his sons, who wanted to take Benjamin with them into Egypt, "If harm befall him by the way in which ye go, then will ye bring down my gray hairs with sorrow to the grave . . ." (Genesis 42:38). This passage shows that, even thousands of years ago, the influence of emotions on the body's functions was already taken to be self-evident. There is no reason for us to feel sorry for ourselves because of all the "terrible stress that modern civilization imposes on us." We should try to analyze the problem more rationally.

There are many emotional influences on the body, familiar to everyone. We get red in the face with shame or embarrassment; we grow pale with fright; stagefright causes "butterflies in the stomach"; sorrow will make us lose our appetite; excitement will make our heart pound rapidly, or miss a beat; in the polygraph test palm sweat is taken as a sign of lying; etc. These are only a few examples.

Some Near Eastern nomadic tribes have an interesting way of "proving" the guilt of suspects of serious crimes. They heat a pan over the fire till it is very hot; then the accused is made to pass his tongue quickly over the inner surface of the pan. If his tongue is burned, he is the culprit. If not, he is pronounced innocent. Probably this custom is based upon the observation that fright arrests saliva secretion, causing dryness of the mouth and tongue, a sensation everyone has surely experienced. In this test it is assumed that an innocent man is not afraid, his saliva flows normally, and therefore his tongue will not stick to the pan.

What is seen here is not the influence of various emotional experiences on psychological or mental processes but rather, their direct influence on the proper function and well-being of the body. In contrast to stress, which gives rise to a well-defined physiological reaction, no matter what the particular cause may be, the reactions enumerated above differ from each other according to what provoked each of them. There are situations in which emotions have a detrimental effect and may even endanger life. Here is an impressive case: A man was put on trial for embezzling money. Throughout the trial he was calm, because he knew that the prosecution had no evidence against him. The only person who could supply the evidence was his partner, who—of course—would never tell. The trial neared its end when the prosecution announced a surprise witness, whereupon the partner appeared in the door. The accused collapsed immediately, of what was diagnosed as a myocardial infarction (heart attack).

Another case: An elderly woman was hospitalized for cancer. The family was told that there was no immediate danger to her life. On the third day of hospitalization her husband wheeled her to the X-ray department for examination and waited for her outside. While being examined, she died suddenly. When the news was brought to her husband, he collapsed and died on the spot.

These two instances illustrate the danger of certain strong emotions. Frustration, sense of personal betrayal, death of a close person, severe insult, great anger, and the like—all these have not only serious psychological impact, but may influence organic functions detrimentally.

A New Attitude

There is no way to avoid difficult situations such as those described above. Doctors', and others', admonitions to cardiac patients to avoid excitement are not very effective. Nobody *wants* to experience tragedy, but this is what life has in store for many of us. Since we cannot run away from sorrow and frustration, perhaps we can react to them differently, by changing our attitude.

In a ten-year prospective study of 10,000 government employees in Israel, one puzzling finding was that religious people had fewer heart attacks than nonreligious. Similar studies in other countries produced the same findings. The difference could not be explained by any of the known variables and is still not understood. But one can speculate. Is it possible that religious believers are less vulnerable because their set of values is different? Perhaps they are more resigned, believing that things are destined to happen, and they do not react to them as if they were a personal affront? Perhaps their attitude of mind makes it easier for them to accept difficult and exasperating situations that produce heart attacks?

Other people appear to be helped by various forms of meditation or the like. The evidence that meditation has a blood-pressure-lowering effect is questionable, but perhaps it helps to promote overall serenity and detachment.

Obviously, nobody will become religious because this may somewhat lessen his or her chances of having a heart attack; nor is meditation everybody's cup of tea. Religion and meditation are being discussed here because they have effects that are documented and must be dealt with in the context of physiological influences of emotions. If it is true that attitude can mitigate dangerous influences on the body's functions in moments of difficulty and calamity, the fact has an obvious implication for all of us. It means that the physiological impact on the human organism of emotionally difficult situations depends, at least partly, on how we react to them. To a certain degree emotional attitude can be *influenced* by reason.

CHAPTER FOUR

Nutrition and Health

Survival

The first act of a human being after birth is to cry for food. The process of gathering enough food was mankind's main concern for many thousands of years, and it still is in much of the world. To get enough food, not to die of starvation, not to be undernourished, these constitute the first and foremost instinct of survival. It is not surprising that accumulation of food plays a pivotal role in motivating human behavior. It has to a large extent established mankind's attitude toward other people, animals, plants, and the world in general.

It is not easy to reconstruct the composition of the diets consumed by ancient societies. From what is known of some Stone-Age societies living today, it can be deduced that people ate what was available. First, they simply gathered food; later, they developed tools for hunting and fishing; finally, they learned to grow plants and tame animals.

Surprisingly, people have managed to survive on all kinds of diets, completely different, but often very monotonous and consisting of very few items. Eskimos, in their primitive stage, lived almost exclusively on seal and fish and some caribou meat. Some tribes in Africa ate mainly yam (a starchy root of some climbing vines) and fruit. For others, the main staple was cereals of one kind or another. For primitive peoples, the pattern is similar everywhere: There is one main staple, while some other foods are known but not easily obtainable.

Taste

In the process of human evolution, man had to learn what he should and should not eat. In other words, he had to eliminate plants containing very little edible substance or none at all. The same applied to poisonous plants and toxic living organisms. In the course of this process of elimination, man learned what was good for him and what was harmful.

Concomitantly, taste developed. In all societies some foods are more appreciated and desired than others. People usually like to eat what they have learned to eat in their childhood. Indians and Mexicans, for instance, eat very spicy hot foods and enjoy them, whereas most Europeans could not taste these foods without getting tears in their eyes. There is no doubt that our tastes are largely formed in childhood by the kind of food that is available in a given society.

Folklore and Religion

Naturally, food had—and still has—enormous influence on human folklore and superstition, and vice versa. It was thought in earlier times that our behavior and actions were influenced by what we eat. For thousands of years mankind believed in the magical and pharmacological properties of food. In every primitive society there were and are special foods and concoctions for all occasions of life, including disease. Love potions are perhaps the best known and varied, though quite often they contain ingreients such as animal testicles. Animal hearts were frequently sought by fighters and hunters to give them courage. Those are just two examples. Even in our times in Western society, some of these beliefs *still* persist.

Food is of such physiological importance that it could of course not be ignored by religions. Many religions have quite a lot to say on the subject of food. They define what is allowed to be eaten and what is forbidden, and even lay down rules as to how food should be prepared, as well as what should be eaten when.

Appetite

Appetite influences to a large extent what we eat, especially in the societies where food supply is abundant. Appetite should not be confused with hunger, which is physiologically and psychologically a completely different sensation. Appetite tells us, given the choice, what to eat, and how much.

To illustrate this point let us imagine a group of, say, one hundred people at an elegant buffet dinner. The tables are loaded with many kinds of different and attractive dishes. Everybody takes a plate and fills it according to taste and appetite. I affirm that no two guests will eat precisely the same things, qualitatively or quantitatively—if second helpings and leftovers on the plate are taken into consideration.

Now Science, Too

What we eat, how much we eat, and at what time, are determined by the factors detailed above. For ages man has eaten for survival and pleasure. Even today, we do not eat because of scientific or medical considerations, although lately preoccupation with health has had more and more influence on our menus. As will be explained in detail later, a "scientific diet" does not exist. It would be impossible to formulate a definite diet, based on scientifically established and proven facts, determining what and how much any individual should eat in order to be healthy. The best we can do at present is to give an outline to the general public as to which foods should be avoided, which should be eaten in smaller quantities, and which can be consumed in any quantities desired.

The science of nutrition — as opposed to the science of food preparation — is relatively new. It evolved in the nineteenth century. At that time, rice was the major staple food in the Far East. It was discovered that a severe disease called beri-beri affected only people living in areas where polished rice was eaten; that is, rice from which the outer hull was removed. Together with the hull, the germinal part containing vitamin B_1 was discarded. Beri-beri was found to be a vitamin-deficiency disease. The discovery that minute quantities of certain substances in food made a difference between health and disease gave great impetus to nutritional science, igniting the imaginations of scientists and public. Scientists set out to analyze food items carefully to find out what substances each of them contained that are necessary to our health. Other vitamins were discovered, their values investigated, their sources revealed — and our daily needs for them calculated. Eventually, nearly all foods were studied. Their contents of carbohydrates, fats, proteins, vitamins, and minerals were noted. People were told what to eat in order to obtain all they needed to grow and be healthy. This was the *positive period of nutritional science,* and it led to the virtual elimination of nutritional deficiency in Europe and North America.

With the advent of the affluent society, things changed, because food is now potentially available in unlimited quantities to practically everybody. Protein and vitamin deficiency — responsible for most diseases of malnutrition — have virtually disappeared. In many countries, deficiency diseases, as they are called, can today be found only in medical textbooks or in cases of mentally unbalanced people, alcoholics, or the like.

Some diseases, however, have clearly increased in incidence. Among these, arteriosclerosis, which is responsible for 50 percent of human mortality, is the most important. Among other diseases whose incidence has increased are dental decay (caries), appendicitis, constipation, and ulcerative colitis. At this point, nutritional science entered a new phase: *the negative phase.* Today each food item is again being thoroughly investigated, this time to determine whether it contains substances *harmful* to our health. People are now being told, mainly, what is "bad for you" — which items should be banned and which restricted.

The Magic Triangle

We have seen that foods eaten in various societies differ, to a very great extent. However, when total food intake is computed, it turns out that the percentage of fats, carbohydrates, and protein is remarkably similar in all societies, with only a few exceptions.

Let us draw a triangle. The upper angle is marked "P" for protein, the left one "CH" for carbohydrates, and the right one "F" for fats. The relative composition of an individual's or group's or nation's food intake is inserted in the triangle and marked by a dot. A dot on the P angle indicates that only protein is eaten. If no protein at all is eaten, but only fat and carbohydrates, we would put the dot on the bottom line, opposite the letter P. This shows that protein intake is zero. The same goes for the other two angles. An equal amount of all three, would be marked by a dot in the center of the triangle, equidistant from all three angles. Primitive societies on the verge of malnutrition consume only about 8 percent protein. Of the remaining 92 percent of food in their diet, two-thirds consists of carbohydrates. This is marked in the lower left corner of the small rectangle inside the triangle.

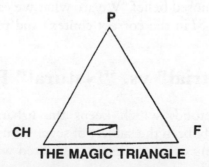

THE MAGIC TRIANGLE

In the affluent society, the protein content in the menu is generally doubled, to about 16 percent. Fat and carbohydrates are eaten in more or less equal quantities, with a little more fat. The percentage difference between the two types of diets is rather small. It is denoted by the arrow spanning from the lower-left corner to the upper-right corner of the small rectangle. This is an interesting finding, showing that in spite of unlimited availability of food in the affluent society, the relative composition of the diet is not very different from that of the poorer societies. This is probably an indication of the body's basic physiological needs.

Small as the difference may be, in relative terms, in reality it is very marked. First, qualitatively: The protein and fat consumed in poor societies derives mainly from plants, whereas in the affluent society it is mainly of animal origin, such as meat, eggs, and dairy products. There is also a major quantitative difference. Whereas in many poor nations calorie intake may not exceed 1400 per person per day, in the rich ones it is almost double that amount. Eight percent protein of 1400 calories is about 28 grams, while 16 percent of 2600 calories is about 100 grams. The same goes for fat: 30 percent of 1400 calories in the poor countries is about 40 grams of fat, while 42 percent of 2600 calories make about 120 grams.

This difference is crucial. It assures growth to the genetic maximum, freedom from food-deficiency diseases, increase in blood proteins, which boosts resistance to tuberculosis and other chronic infections, and finally an average life expectancy of about 70 years. On the other hand, it exposes us to greater risk of other diseases, which usually take their toll later in life: the so-called diseases of civilization. There can be little doubt that the time-honored belief "We are what we eat" cannot be denied if *understood* in the correct context and proportion.

"Industrial" vs. "Natural" Food

Mass-produced food, which keeps the urban population supplied, has lately been the subject of severe abuse. Such food is accused of being over-processed, tampered with, tasteless, "unnatural," containing too many additives—and so on. Where is yesteryear's tasty "natural" food? We have probably all heard fond reminiscences of the good and wholesome food in the days of our grandparents.

The truth is far removed from this nostalgia. Never in the history of mankind has food supply been so abundant and so varied as today. Never before could so many different items from faraway continents be purchased, at reasonable prices, to enrich our diet and please our palates. Never has food been so hygienically packed and subject to such supervision of quality and standards. Let us not forget that at the beginning of this century, large-scale freezing, frozen transportation, and commercial and home refrigerators were virtually nonexistent. Supermarkets did not exist until recent decades. The time needed to make the journey from producer to consumer took longer than is good for unrefrigerated food. Consequently, in the past, foods were not always in good condition by the time they reached the kitchen. Infections were more common. Unpasteurized milk, even when boiled, was not always safe, and certainly not very tasty.

To preserve food for longer periods of time, it was often packed in huge quantities of salt. Additives for coloring, consistency, and preservation were part of the deal, most of these processes unsupervised as to quality and quantity. "Exotic foods" from foreign countries were often very expensive and hard to come by. Some items were available on the market only for very short seasons.

How can all this be compared to the kind of food that one can purchase today at the neighborhood supermarket? Beyond a doubt, food is by far tastier, healthier, more hygienic than the "natural" food of 70 or more years ago. Freezing and other modern methods of food preservation have to a great extent eliminated geographical and seasonal limitations, increasing choice and availability.

As to the food additives used for preservation, consistency, and coloring, many are not new, and have been traditionally used for a long time—in some cases, hundreds of years. Others have been introduced more recently. Most have been investigated and tested thoroughly by the Food and Drug

Administration of the United States government, as well as by food scientists, and found harmless. Obviously, periodic testing, repeated investigation, and control of production and product must go on indefinitely. This will assure the customer that what he buys and eats does not contain harmful substances, for in this respect public pressure will certainly not relent.

It should, however, be remembered that possible harmful effects usually depend on the quantity of food consumed. This is especially true for food that has additives. If one is not a food faddist, subsisting only on a limited number of foods, but instead on a menu consisting of many varied foods, possible harm to health is greatly reduced. As in so much that is related to health, quantity is of major importance. Very often it is not a question of yes or no, but of how much.

The Composition of Food

The scientific classification of food is basically simple. The three major components of food are carbohydrates, fats, and proteins. A fourth group are the "essential" nutrients: vitamins, minerals, and a limited amount of protein (see below). The word "essential" denotes substances that the body cannot produce from other substances that are ingested, but that must be obtained in their final form from outside.

Most of the food we eat is converted into energy, which the body needs in order to perform its functions. The major part of this energy is expended in muscular work. We can obtain the required energy from any quantitative mixture of carbohydrates, fats, and proteins, and one can be substituted for the other. The essential nutrients are not used to produce energy but are necessary for various metabolic functions. Unlike the foods we use for energy, they cannot be replaced by other substances. Each of these is needed by the body for certain function and usually in small quantities. Deficiency of these nutrients seriously impairs the body's functions, resulting in disease. Lack of vitamins can give rise to avitaminoses, which may be fatal and are widespread in underdeveloped countries. Iron deficiency may cause anemia, iodine deficiency, thyroid disease, etc.

There are two more components in our food: (1) water, which is essential to life and is contained in most foods, and (2) roughage, or dietary fiber, which is the unabsorbed part of the foods we eat. During the positive phase of nutritional science, fiber had been neglected and considered unimportant, even unnecessary. Lately, however, it has attracted attention and assumed its proper place in nutritional science.

Digestion and Absorption

The food we eat is cut into small pieces by the teeth. In the chewing process it is mixed with saliva, which contains some digestive enzymes. The food is then swallowed, and is processed in the gastrointestinal tract. Usually the food is composed of large molecules. Enzymes of the digestive juices break them up into smaller components, fit for absorption into the wall of the digestive tract and from there into the blood. In the stomach digestive juices operate in a very acid milieu, starting to break up proteins. From here the food mixture moves into the duodenum, or upper part of the small intestine. Here digestive juices from the pancreas are added, as well as bile from the liver, which facilitates fat digestion.

In the small intestine more digestive juices are secreted and their enzymes act upon all components of food (carbohydrates, fats, proteins), splitting them into small molecules, which are readily absorbed. The inner lining of the small intestine has many folds, producing an absorption area of some 100 square feet. Here everything is absorbed into the bloodstream and carried to the liver for processing. In the large bowel the remaining water and salts are absorbed, and feces are formed. These weigh about 7 to 10 ounces daily, and contain the unabsorbable fiber as well as some water.

The total quantity of digestive juices secreted daily into the intestinal tract is about 8 to 9 quarts. These, together with the food and beverages ingested, may amount to some 12 to 15 quarts, or even more when we drink a lot. All this, except the very small quantity excreted with the feces, is absorbed by the body daily. Quite a remarkable feat!

Absorption of food, except for fiber and some minerals, is complete. Only minuscule quantities of digestible food are excreted in the feces. This is one of the most efficiently functioning systems of the body. It does not make any difference whether we eat slowly or rapidly, chew properly or not, eat hot or cold food, cooked or raw—absorption proceeds anyway.

Carbohydrates

Carbohydrates are made of three elements: carbon, oxygen, and hydrogen. The basic molecule has six carbon atoms. There are three simple sugars or, as they are called chemically, monosaccharides (equal to one molecule of sugar): glucose, galactose, and fructose. All three have the same basic composition and caloric value, but are digested by different enzymes. Yeast, for example, can digest glucose and produce alcohol, but it cannot attack galactose, which is contained in milk.

Usually we do not eat sugar in the form of mono-saccharides but as disaccharides, consisting of two molecules of simple sugar, or as polysaccharides, chains containing many molecules of simple sugar (monosaccharide). There are three disaccharides: maltose, lactose, and sucrose. Maltose (glucose + glucose) is found in malt, sugar beets, and other substances; lactose (glucose + galactose) in milk and milk products; sucrose (glucose + fructose) in sugar cane and many fruits. Refined sugar (the sugar served at the table and used for cooking and baking) is made up of these disaccharides.

However, most of the carbohydrates we consume are in the form of starch, which is a polysaccharide also known as complex carbohydrate. Starch is composed of hundreds of molecules of glucose. It is the major component of cereals (wheat, millet, oats, rye, corn, rice, barley, etc.) and of potatoes. It was and still is the most important staple of the human race. As we have seen, it accounts for about 60 percent of the calories consumed in primitive societies and about a quarter of the calories in affluent ones. Table 1 lists foods rich in carbohydrates.

TABLE 1
CARBOHYDRATE-RICH FOOD
(grams per 100 grams or 3⅓ ounces)

	Calories	Carbohydrate	Fat	Protein
Sugar	400	100	—	—
Cornflour	350	82	—	—
Rice	360	87	1	7
Noodles	370	80	2	13
Flour, wheat	330	80	1	10
Bread, white	235	50	2	8
Bread, wholemeal	215	42	3	9
Potatoes	60	16	—	2
Cornflakes	370	85	2	9
Matzo	385	85	2	11
Legumes	300	50	1	22

As for absorption from the gastrointestinal tract into the bloodstream, there is a great difference between starch and sugar. All carbohydrates are absorbed as monosaccharides and partly as disaccharides. Sugars are ingested as disaccharides, so that only one bond linking the two monosaccharides must be opened in the digestive tract, a task rapidly performed. Consequently, sugar is absorbed very rapidly. Furthermore, sugar is one of only three substances that can be partly absorbed by the stomach, even before it reaches the small intestine (the other two are water and alcohol). This rapid absorption can introduce a large quantity of sugar into the blood in a short time, which can strain the body's metabolic pathways. It is assumed that this rapid absorption enhances obesity, and is possibly in other ways harmful. It is definitely bad for diabetics, who do not have the means to deal with large quantities of sugar at one time. This is why diabetic patients are told not to eat sugar or sugar-containing foods.

Starch, on the other hand, is broken down slowly. It is

arranged in long chains of monosaccharides, which are broken down gradually in the small intestine; thereby, the amount of sugar released into the blood stream at any one time is small. Furthermore, carbohydrates of the cereal and legume families are usually surrounded by fiber, which hinders the action of the digestive enzymes and delays the process of absorption. The difference between sugars and starches lies in the way they are absorbed. While sugar is absorbed in a matter of minutes, the same quantity of starch needs several hours to be totally absorbed.

Sugar

Sugar is extracted in refineries from beets or sugar cane, and is then processed into crystalline form. This familiar white substance comes in the form of cubes, granules, or powder, and contains 100 percent sugar. In many countries brown sugar is available which is also refined—but not completely. It contains about 95 percent refined sugar and some water. There is no significant difference between the two. In other countries, brown sugar is completely refined sugar, with caramel and flavoring added for coloring and taste.

Sugar is added to hot and cold beverages, most breakfast cereals, candy, chocolate, cakes, desserts, ice cream, and practically everything that must have a sweet taste. Sugar, in its refined form, is a relatively new product. In the Bible, the Promised Land was described as "the land of milk and honey." It says honey because refined sugar was nonexistent at the time. People ate honey, or sugar cane, or extracts of dates and carobs. When sugar was first produced commercially, it immediately became a tremendous success. Love at first sight! Its consumption has increased steadily throughout the world. In the United States, the yearly consumption per person is now about 132 pounds, which is about two pounds and a half weekly, up from 118 pounds yearly in 1975!

Many physicians, nutritionists, and researchers view sugar with misgivings. It is believed to be instrumental in promoting some of the so-called "diseases of civilization"—notably, heart

disease, obesity, dental decay (caries), and possibly diabetes —
though none of these charges, except caries, have been proven.
It is generally agreed that the consumption of refined sugar
should be curtailed.

Can this be done? This is one of the few problems concerning food in which the answer is unequivocally yes. One
can certainly subsist without refined sugar. Nobody ate refined
sugar at all until a few hundred years ago; a person can live
to very old age and be healthy without ever touching it.
Cutting down on refined sugar or abstaining from it
completely can unhesitatingly be recommended, because a lack
of it will cause no harm.

But *should* we totally renounce the pleasure of the sweet
taste that we love so much? Certainly not. There are several
sugar substitutes now on the market: saccharine (300 times as
sweet as sugar), aspartame or Nutrasweet (180 times sweeter),
and in some countries cyclamate (30 times sweeter) as well,
which, by the way, is the tastiest of the three. Eighty-five
percent of people cannot distinguish cyclamate from sugar if
it is used in the right concentration. In beverages and many
foods, these sweeteners can substitute for sugar completely.
In other foods, they can do so partly, reducing sugar consumption to a large extent. In reasonable quantities, artificial
sweeteners cause no damage and do not enhance the development of cancer (see pages 146–149). They are a blessing for
the many people who find it difficult to do without the sweet
taste but do not want to use sugar because of its high caloric
value. One gram of sugar provides four calories and one
teaspoon twenty. Sweeteners are certainly a very great help to
diabetics, who can now eat many kinds of sugarless sweets.
Several more sugar substitutes are now in various stages of
research and development.

Honey

Honey is a viscous solution of mono-and disaccharides in
water, containing about 80 percent sugar. Vitamin and mineral
content is very low and there is practically no protein. It differs
from refined sugar on two accounts: its special taste, preferred

by many, and its price, which is remarkably higher than sugar (when its price is not artificially maintained).

The claim that honey is in any way superior to sugar is completely unfounded. It is not "healthier"; nor is it permitted for diabetics any more than is sugar. It certainly does not have any healing effects or preventive action against any disease. It is not a sugar substitute; it is — sugar.

Fats

Fats, are composed only of carbon, oxygen, and hydrogen, but in different proportions than is the case with carbohydrates. Their main components are fatty acids. Each three fatty acids are attached to a glycerin molecule, forming a triglyceride. Most of the fat that we consume is in the form of triglycerides.

Fatty acids are composed of chains of carbon atoms. To each carbon atom one or two atoms of hydrogen are attached. At one end of the chain there is an organic acid, in which two oxygen atoms are incorporated. There are many different kinds of fatty acids. Some have a short chain, just a few carbon atoms, others, a very long one, of about 20 carbon atoms or more. What is important in modern medicine, however, is not the length of the chain but the number of hydrogen atoms attached to the carbon chain. In the so-called *saturated* fatty acids, there is the maximum possible number of hydrogen atoms attached to each of the carbon atoms. In other words, "saturated" means that the fatty acid is completely saturated by hydrogen (see chart "Central Part of Fatty Acids").

CENTRAL PART OF FATTY ACIDS

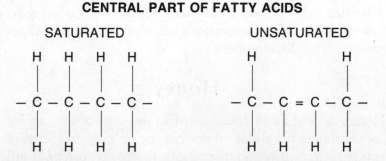

Each carbon atom has 4 arms to form bonds with other atoms.

In the unsaturated fatty acids, some carbon atoms are attached to each other by double bonds, and consequently the number of hydrogen atoms is smaller (see figure). When there is only one double bond, we speak of a *mono-unsaturated* acid; when there are more, of a *poly-unsaturated* acid.

It has been proven that a diet rich in saturated fatty acids raises the blood cholesterol level, promoting the development of arteriosclerosis. The total daily fat intake in the affluent society averages 120 grams, four to five times that in under-developed countries. The fat in most foods preferred by Americans and Europeans is, unfortunately, saturated— presenting us with a major health problem.

The fat in beef, lamb, pork, poultry, meat products such as sausage, milk and its derivatives such as butter, cheese, and cream, most margarines, and eggs is saturated. Most liquid fats obtained or derived from plants are unsaturated: soybean oil, sesame oil, cottonseed oil, sunflower oil, corn oil, safflower oil are poly-unsaturated. Olive oil is mono-unsaturated. On the other hand coconut oil is the most saturated of all fats. Peanuts also contain saturated fat, while other nuts and almonds contain unsaturated oil. Fish oil is mostly unsaturated.

Table 2 lists fat-rich substances.

TABLE 2
FAT-RICH FOOD
(grams per 100 grams or 3⅓ ounces)

	Calories	Carbohydrate	Fat	Protein
Oil	900	—	100	—
Margarine	730	—	81	—
Butter	740	—	82	—
Beef, fat	640	—	67	9
Almonds	560	4	53	17
Peanuts	570	9	50	24
Walnuts	525	5	51	11
Sweet Cream	330	2	35	2
Pork, average	340	—	32	14
Beef, average	280	—	24	16
Beef, lean	125	—	5	20

TABLE 2, continued

	Calories	Carbohydrate	Fat	Protein
Cheese, processed	310	—	25	22
Eggs	150	—	11	12
Milk, whole	65	5	4	3

Cholesterol is not a fat; it belongs to a group called lipoids, meaning fat-like substances. It is not soluble in water, but only in fat solvents such as alcohol, ether, etc. Cholesterol has been identified in the arteriosclerotic plaques that form in the blood vessels and has been linked with the development of arteriosclerosis (page 000). It has been found that the higher the blood-cholesterol level, the greater the risk of heart attacks. The blood level of cholesterol, however, is influenced in addition to genetics mainly by the saturated fat contained in our diet and to a much lesser extent by the cholesterol consumed. The relationship between fat ingestion and arteriosclerosis and what can be done about it, is discussed on page 000.

It is important not to mix up *blood cholesterol levels* with the amount of *cholesterol in our food*. Cholesterol is present only in animal products and their derivatives (meat, milk, eggs). Many food producers advertise: "Contains no cholesterol." This however, does not mean too much. The important thing is to find out whether the food you want to buy contains much saturated fat. For example: Shrimp and other seafood items are relatively high in cholesterol but contain almost no saturated fat. A study has found that ingestion of shrimp does not increase blood cholesterol levels.

Proteins

Proteins are the building blocks of the living organism. In addition to carbon, oxygen, and hydrogen—of which fats and carbohydrates are composed—proteins contain 16 percent nitrogen and some sulphur. Proteins are chains of amino acids.

There are 22 different amino acids, all of them with the same characteristic structure. The central part of the molecule is specific to each one of them, while at the one end there is an organic acid (COOH) and at the other an amino-group (NH2). The acid group of one amino acid links with the amino group of another amino group. In this way long chains are formed—the proteins (see charts "Composition of Amino Acids" and "Composition of Chains of Proteins").

COMPOSITION OF AMINO ACIDS

NH2 ——	C.P.	—— COOH
Amino	Central	Organic
group	part	acid

In all amino acids there is at one end an amino group and at the other the organic acid. Each of the 22 amino acids differs from the others in the composition of the central part (C.P.).

COMPOSITION OF CHAINS OF PROTEINS

–NH2–CP1–COOH–NH2–CP2–COOH–NH2–CP3–COOH–

Protein chains are formed from amino acids, which are always linked to each other in the same way: The amino group (NH2) of one amino acids attaches itself to the organic acid (COOH) of its neighbor.

Just as with 26 letters one can form an innumerable amount of words, nature has composed from 22 amino acids an astonishingly large number of different protein chains, each of a particular composition. Each species in nature has its own specific protein formula. The protein of beef, for example, differs from the protein of the human body in the number and sequence of the amino acids it contains. Human protein differs from that of corn or rice, etc. The difference is not only in the number of the various amino acids in the chain, but also in the way they are arranged within the chain. Let us take for example, part of the chain of proteins of two hypothetical species. If for simplicity's sake, we assign a number instead of the name of each amino acid, we obtain the following sequences:

Series 1: . . . 1–7–7–13–2–2–8–8–10–12–8–8–1–8–7 . . .

Series 2: . . . 13–7–9–3–21–21–15–5–4–4–18–9–21–8 . . .

When we eat protein, the chains are *broken* by enzymes in our digestive tract, and the amino acids are freed. Each one is absorbed into the blood separately and carried to the liver and other cells, where human protein chains are built from the raw material. Most amino acids can be produced by the body, though only from other amino acids already *ingested*. Nine amino acids, however, are "essential" ones—meaning that our body cannot form them but has to obtain them from the outside.

Which proteins are best for us? Obviously, those that contain essential amino acids in the same or similar proportion as contained in the formula of human protein. From this point of view, cow's milk and egg white are best—at least theoretically. In practice, the same result can be obtained in another way, even if eggs and cow's milk are not included in the diet.

Let us go back to our two hypothetical protein sequences, assuming that amino acids 21, 9, 10, and 12 are "essential." If we restrict ourselves to protein of series 1, we shall be deficient in amino acids 21 and 9. If we restrict ourselves to series 2, we shall lack the essential amino acids 10 and 12. But if we eat proteins of both species, we shall get all the essential amino acids we need because the series will complement each other. The conclusion is clear: We must eat many different protein sources to be sure that we get all the necessary essential amino acids.

In the affluent society, however, this consideration is also mainly theoretical, because we are ingesting a great surplus of protein. Children need about 1 gram of protein per 1 kilogram (2.2 lbs.) of body weight. Grownups can very well manage on 0.5 grams per kilogram, and less. This means that in practice an individual weighing 80 kg. (176 lbs.) needs about 40 grams (one and one-third ounces) of protein daily. In the United

States and in Western European countries, average protein consumption is 100 to 120 grams per day, two to three times the required amount.

Table 3 lists protein-rich foods. Several aspects are striking. First, no food contains more than 25 percent protein except soy beans. Second protein-rich foods of animal origin, such as eggs, milk, cheese, and meat but not sea fish, contain much saturated fat while nuts and almonds are high in proteins and unsaturated fat. Third, the vegetable family of legumes—i.e., beans, lentils, soy beans, peas, chick peas, etc.—have a high protein content, are rich in carbohydrates, and are low in fat (except soy beans). Fourth, it is remarkable and often overlooked that the cereal family and its products, such as flour, bread, noodles, cornflakes, oats, etc., contain about 10 percent protein, so that in addition to supplying the body with carbohydrates, these too are an important source of protein.

TABLE 3
PROTEIN-RICH FOOD
(grams per 100 grams or 3⅓ ounces)

	Calories	Carbohydrate	Fat	Protein
Soy, flour	450	24	24	3
Wheat, flour	330	80	1	10
Cheese, processed	310	—	25	22
Peanuts	570	9	50	24
Almonds	560	4	53	17
Walnuts	525	5	51	11
Peas, dried	290	50	1	22
Lentils, dried	300	53	1	24
Beans, dried	270	50	1	20
Cheese, white, lean	90	1	—	22
Beef, average	280	—	24	16
Pork, average	340	—	32	14
Fish: cod, haddock	76	—	1	10
Eggs	150	—	11	12
Noodles	370	80	2	12
Matzo	385	85	2	11
Bread	235	50	2	9
Milk	65	5	4	3

In summary, protein is an extremely important component in our nutritional requirements. In some underdeveloped countries, protein deficiency is widespread and causes diseases. However, in our society one glance at the table of the protein-rich foods we eat is enough to convince us that there is no protein problem! As a matter of fact, we are getting two or three times what we need. Our main problem seems to be the high saturated-fat content of protein-rich food of animal origin. Ways to cut down on the fat are detailed on pages 18–19.

Vitamins

Vitamins are substances essential for the proper functioning of our metabolism. Many physiological processes in the living organism cannot proceed properly without the presence of vitamins. Their absence causes severe deficiency diseases.

I do not intend to enumerate here all the vitamins, nor to list the foods that contain them. Such an undertaking would be superfluous in a book on health in the affluent society. Vitamins are substances that the body needs in minute quantities. It is easy to get enough of them if one eats a more or less normal diet. The truth of the matter is that in the affluent society vitamin deficiency can be found only in cases of eccentric food faddists, in severe alcoholics, in people who do not eat because of mental disorders, or when there is disease—in which latter case the body's capacity to process the substances into which the vitamins are incorporated, is impaired.

The minimal daily requirement for vitamins, as outlined by the World Health Organization and by the U.S. health authorities, is easily met, and usually exceeded, in a normal diet. Nevertheless, today there is a great deal of preoccupation with vitamins. The notion that minute quantities of a vitamin may make the difference between health and disease appeals to the imagination of doctors and public alike. And let us not forget that powerful drug companies discovered long ago that vitamin production can be a gold mine. Whereas drugs are sold to sick people, and usually for a limited period of time, vitamins, if well advertised, can be sold to the entire population throughout life.

Under these circumstances it is not surprising that time and again we are being told by various non-medical sources that high doses, and sometimes very high doses, of vitamins are health-promoting, prolong life, prevent a variety of diseases, have great healing effects, etc. None of this has ever been scientifically proven. Attempts to verify certain claims, by scientifically controlled experiments, have always been negative. There is no evidence whatsoever that high doses of vitamin C can prevent or shorten a cold, nor have other claims been substantiated. They seem to belong to the realm of wishful thinking, mythology, or superstition.

Most vitamins (except A and D) are, fortunately, water-soluble; and any excess is excreted in the urine without causing harm. Cases of vitamin D overdoses have been described. *Very high doses* of water-soluble vitamins can sometimes be harmful; even damaging effects of vitamin C overdoses have been reported.

It is biologically unsound to think that good health will be promoted by very high doses of vitamins, in excess of what are found in a normal diet. The human body is made up of substances that are present on earth and its basic needs are adapted to the available water, air, and food in quantities fairly readily attainable from nature. Any mutation causing the body to require exotic substances not easily available from the environment could not exist for long. It is unthinkable that a species would evolve that requires certain substances in quantities unobtainable by normal nutrition. A race needing such things would have become extinct a long time ago.

It is worth knowing that cooking, baking, frying, and other processing of food does not usually decrease vitamin content by more than 30 percent. Vitamin C is an exception, because about 50 percent of it is destroyed by heating, and it is therefore best obtained from raw fruits and vegetables.

Minerals

Our body contains about sixty different elements. Oxygen, nitrogen, hydrogen, carbon, sulphur, phosphorus, and a few other enumerated below are present in large quantities and are essential. Most of the others are found in the body in minuscule quantities and probably do not play any significant role in our metabolism. Calcium and phosphorus are deposited in the bones, giving them their hardness and strength. Sodium, chloride, potassium, and magnesium are important components of the extra- and intracellular fluids. Iodine is essential for hormone production in the thyroid gland. Iron is part of hemoglobin, the substance contained in red blood cells; it carries oxygen to the tissues. Other substances that are related to the function of various tissues and organs are fluoride, manganese, copper, and zinc. These elements are usually found in sufficient quantities in food and their supply poses virtually no problem. A few more problematic elements will be discussed below:

Iodine

The sea is rich in iodine, and since most of the earth was at some time or other covered by sea, iodine is present in the ground and in the plants that grow on it. In some high mountain ranges, like the Himalayas and the Alps, which were never covered by the sea and to a lesser extent in other countries, iodine deficiency has produced cases of hypothyroid goiters. Therefore, some countries, including the United States, have required iodine addition to table salt. Today this problem hardly exists. Food in the affluent society is brought from many areas, including faraway countries. Even people living in iodine-poor areas are now getting enough of this mineral.

Iron

Iron-deficiency anemia occurs frequently, especially in women, who lose blood during menstruation. During pregnancy much of a mother's iron is transferred to the fetus. But iron deficiency is not due to a lack of iron in the food. Normally, we must have about 10 milligrams of iron daily in our food (of which only 1 to 2 mgs. can be absorbed).

TABLE 4
IRON CONTENT OF FOOD
(milligrams per 100 grams, or 3⅓ ounces)

Pecans	2.5
Oats	4.5
Peanuts	2
Potatoes, flour	5.5
Almonds	4.5
Spinach	3.5
Walnuts	2
Peas, dried	5.5
Sunflower seeds	7
Chick peas, dried	7
Lentils, dried	7
Eggs	2.5
Eggs, yolk	6.5
Soy bean, flour	10
Beans, dried	7
Apricots, dried	4.5
Raisins	2.5
Figs, dried	4
Cocoa, powder	13
Chocolate, bitter	4.5
Bread	2.5
Coffee, instant	5
Pizza (regular)	4
Beef	3
Beef, liver	10.5
Turkey	4
Sardines	4
Sausages	2

Table 4 lists the iron content of various foods. It shows that practically everyone eats more than 10 mg. of iron daily.

Our problem is absorption. I stated previously that our small intestine is perfectly adjusted to its task and that it absorbs everything. This is true for carbohydrates, fats, and proteins, but not always for iron. Iron absorption decreases during febrile (fever-causing) and other diseases. Even healthy people may have difficulties absorbing enough iron. Though there have been intensive studies, scientists still have not elucidated the factors that inhibit iron absorption.

Since iron deficiency in our society is not due to lack of iron in food, it is useless to eat more iron-rich foods, because this will not raise the blood's iron level. In cases of deficiency, iron intake must be increased up to one-hundred fold to obtain positive results. The only way to do this is to take iron supplements. In some obstinate cases, recourse must be had to injections.

Calcium

Calcium is present in very large quantities in bones and about 10 milligrams per 100 milliliters are found in the bloodstream. Its metabolism is controlled by the hormone of four small endocrine glands, the parathyroids, which are located behind the thyroid gland in the neck. The daily turnover is about 400 to 800 milligrams. We must get this much from food.

The main sources of calcium are milk and milk products, excluding milk fats like butter. A glass of milk contains about 250 mg. calcium. With cheese, 100 gr. (3 ounces) contain between 150 to 300 mg. However, calcium is present in many other foods (see Table 5). Strict vegetarians who do not consume milk or its products do not suffer from calcium deficiency, nor do they seem to be affected by osteoporosis more often than the general population.

TABLE 5
CALCIUM CONTENT OF FOOD
(milligrams per 100 grams or 3⅓ ounces)

Soy, flour	210
Apricots, dried	100
Milk	120
Figs, dried	280
Cheese, hard	400-800
Lemons	110
Yogurt	180
Rhubarb	100
Chocolate, milk	220
Chocolate, drinking	150

TABLE 5, continued

Fruit juice	360
String beans	180
Beans	100
White sauce	140
Baking powder	11,000
Broccoli	100
Vegetables (general)	40
Parsley	330
Onions, spring	140
Spinach, boiled	800
Sardines, canned	550
Shrimps, boiled	320
Fish	15-20
Meat	5-10

Chronically disabled and immobilized people often have a negative calcium balance, meaning that they lose calcium from the bones in larger quantities than it is replaced. In elderly people, especially post-menopausal women, a disease called osteoporosis weakens the bones, and is associated with calcium loss. Increasing calcium intake does not seem to improve the situation. Very high calcium intake, as from tablets, may overload the kidneys with calcium and cause damage to them. The treatment is mainly hormonal.

Salt

Sodium chloride, or plain table salt, is absolutely essential for life. It is a major component of the body fluids, and maintains their osmotic pressure, assuring proper circulation of the fluids in the tissues and the transfer of substances in and out of cells. In ancient times, salt was very precious, especially in countries far removed from the sea. In periods of history it was some-times used as currency. In many countries, salt was a monopoly of king or state until recent times.

The salt level of the body fluids is kept constant by the action of several hormones, and if too much is consumed, the excess will be excreted in the urine. If intake is small, the kidneys will reabsorb into the bloodstream almost all the salt that passes through them.

The quantity of salt eaten varies considerably from one country to another and from one individual to another. In some primitive societies average salt consumption is about 3 grams daily, while in other areas it may reach 15 to 20 grams. Normal Western diets contain between 5 to 15 grams of salt a day. People have very different habits concerning uses of salt. There are three distinct groups: One never adds salt to food and dislikes heavily salted food. The second tastes food first and sometimes adds salt, while the members of the third group always add salt—even without tasting.

Hypertension and Salt

Hypertension, or high blood pressure, is a disease with genetic background, but it is clearly associated with salt intake. In countries where salt content in food is low, hypertension is rarer, and vice versa. In examining groups of people classified according to their salt consumption, it was found that the incidence of hypertensive disorders was higher among those who ate a lot of salt.

The relationship between salt intake and hypertension is not well understood. It may be an inability of some people's kidneys to excrete all the excess salt; it may also be that damage is caused to certain kidney cells when they must excrete much salt.

But not everyone eating a great deal of salt will develop hypertension. Hypertension runs in families and this indicates that there is, rather, a constitutional and genetic predisposition for the disease. A high salt intake may possibly advance the disease in some susceptible individuals.

The connection of salt to hypertension and its other possible harmful effects, such as enhancing arteriosclerosis, has led some researchers and nutritionists to suggest that the whole population should reduce salt intake drastically, to about 3 grams daily or less.

This recommendation is problematic, for several reasons. As has been explained in a previous chapter, man can very well live without refined sugar, but he cannot live without salt.

And in contrast to sugar, there is no good salt substitute on the market; most people find available salt substitutes unacceptable. Finally, we get only a small part of the daily salt intake from the salt shaker! Some salt is present in food in its natural state, but most of it is added during processing or cooking. A diet very low in salt is generally considered to be unpalatable, and people who have to adhere to it, as in cases of heart failure, often suffer severely. In effect, it means doing without many foods that are important in our diet.

Table 6 lists the content of salt in various foods. While most vegetables, fruits, and oils contain less than 25 milligrams per 100 grams, other vegetables such as carrots, cabbage, and beets, have 150 to 250 milligrams per 100 grams. Milk and eggs contain 350 to 400 milligrams per 100 grams. Bread has 800 to 1500 milligrams per 100 grams. Finally, smoked fish, sausage, hard cheese, ketchup, and canned meat contain 2500 to 3500 milligrams per 100 grams. As can be seen in Table 6, just 3 ounces of smoked fish, sausage, or canned meat contain more salt than the recommended "prudent" diet allows.

TABLE 6
SODIUM CONTENT OF FOOD
(milligrams per 100 grams or 3⅓ ounces)

Self-rising flour	350
Rye flour	400
Rice	100
Spaghetti	150
Bread, white	100
Bread, wholemeal	220
All-bran	1,000
Milk	50
Chocolate milk	120
Chocolate drink	250
Butter, salted	870
Margarine, salted	800
Cheese, hard	300–1,400
Eggs	140
Salt	39,000
Olives	2,250

TABLE 6, continued

Tomato juice, canned	230
Baking powder	12,000
Bacon	1,400
Beef	60
Meat, canned	1,000
Chicken	80
Fish, smoked	1,000–1,800

Sodium is 40 percent of cooking salt by weight. To calculate the salt content, multiply by 2.5.

There is little doubt that, by and large, our diet contains considerably less salt than the one our grandparents ate at the beginning of the century. Prior to the modern food-preservation methods, like freezing, many foods were preserved in salt. Meat, vegetables, butter, fish, and many other foods were very heavily salted—to keep them from decaying. It is unknown whether the incidence of hypertension was higher at that time.

It does not seem justifiable to recommend a radical reduction in salt intake for the entire population. For many people it would be a tremendous sacrifice; most people are not harmed by eating 10 to 15 grams of salt a day. And salt may contribute to vitality and energy.

People whose blood pressure is climbing should get treatment, which in many cases might well include salt restriction. Those with a family history of hypertension should have their blood pressure checked once or twice yearly. In case hypertension does appear, treatment can be given immediately so as to prevent complications.

The best advice to the healthy population is to practice some moderation. Most people will not find it difficult to content themselves with 5 to 10 grams of salt daily. This requires only the restriction of very heavily salted foods, and it may be a good idea to be careful with "junk food", which is often very rich in salt. Finally, pressure must be exerted on food producers to use less salt in their products. They will do so as soon as the public demands it. Athletes and people performing strenuous physical work, who consequently sweat heavily, should know that even copious sweating does *not* require any additional salt intake.

Fiber

Before refined sugar became available, dietary sugars were extracted by enzymes of the digestive juices, during digestion in the small bowel from foods containing plant fibers, like dates and figs. Refined sugar to a large extent replaced these fiber-containing plants. This increased the percentage of highly concentrated (high in caloric value and devoid of residue) food in our diet.

Chocolate—extremely high in sugar and fat and easily absorbable without leaving any residue—is a good example of the popularity of concentrated food. White bread is made of flour, from which almost all non-absorbable material has been removed in the process of grinding. Fruit juice is another example of a food with no residue, and there are several more.

Evidence is piling up that the consumption of too much fiberless food is not healthful. Constipation, diseases like diverticulosis, and perhaps even cancer of the rectum may well be associated with lack of roughage in the colon. Furthermore, roughage, consisting mainly of indigestible plant fibers, slows the absorption process in the small intestine, decreasing thereby the sudden massive load on the metabolism caused by rapid absorption of sugars and fats. Fiber delays and decreases to a certain degree, cholesterol absorption; it also seems to be of help in maintaining better blood sugar control in diabetics.

Until recent years, fiber was regarded as superfluous, and was even removed from food if at all possible. It is now generally agreed that fiber is not a nuisance, but, rather, an important ingredient of our diet. It is recommended that we have a fiber intake of up to 40 grams a day.

One can, of course, continue to eat concentrated food and add to the diet one of the commercially available bran preparations that are very high in fibers. But it seems much more logical to do the natural thing and eat a variety of vegetables and fresh and dried fruits, which contain fiber. Certain fruits and vegetables have quite a high fiber content (see Table 7).

TABLE 7
FIBER CONTENT OF FOOD
(grams per 100 grams or 3⅓ ounces)

Bran, wheat	44
All–bran, cereal	27
Oatmeal, raw	7
Cornflakes	2
Wheat, puffed	7
Bread, white	3
Bread, wholemeal	9
Soy, flour	12
Lentils, dried	12
Peas, dried	17
Beans, dried	22
Beans, baked, canned	7
Peanuts	8
Almonds	14
Apricots, dried	24
Prunes, peaches, dried	16
Figs, dried	18
Blackberries	7
Broccoli	28
Cabbage	22
Cauliflower	26
String beans, raw	25

(Many other fruits and vegetables: 1-5.)

The higher the standard of living, the lower the intake of bread. Furthermore, white bread is made of finely ground, fiber-less flour. This is regrettable. Wheat has served for many thousands of years as one of our staple foods. It is relatively high in protein, contains vitamins and minerals in a satisfying mixture, and is devoid of fat. In addition, it is quite high in fiber, if this is not removed in the process of grinding and sifting. Whole grain bread is preferable to white bread, and should regain its proper place on our table.

Legumes

After we have eaten a normal meal containing carbohydrates, the sugar level in the blood increases by about 50 percent and reverts to the base line after approximately two hours. A few years ago, it was found that after eating beans, lentils or other plants of the legume family, the blood level of sugar increased by only 20 percent. Beans, lentils, and other legumes have a carbohydrate content of about 60 percents. Nobody expected legumes to have a different — that is to say, a lesser — effect on our metabolism from any other kind of carbohydrate. It may be due to legumes' greatly delayed absorption rate or to the specific influence of an as-yet-unidentified substance in legumes. See page 20.

Vegetarians and "Naturalists"

Under this heading are groups of individuals who differ widely as to what is included and what is forbidden in their diet. The so-called vegetarians, or lacto-vegetarians, eat everything except meat and fish, their food is cooked, baked, and fried, just as in a normal diet. At the other extreme are the so-called "naturalists," who eat only plant food, to the exclusion of not only meat and fish but eggs, milk and all its products, and also salt and refined sugar, and all sweets, chocolate, and pastries. They eat their food raw. In between these two extremes are many groups who are in several ways more restrictive than the lacto-vegetarians but less so than the outright "naturalists."

The reasons why people adhere to these diets are manifold. Some do it for philosophical or moral reasons; for example, not wanting animals to be slaughtered for food. Others regard such diets as a way of life, a returning from "civilization" to "nature." Others believe that their diet is more healthful than the normal modern diet, that it may heal various afflictions and prevent others. Critical examination of these beliefs is not easy. Many of the extreme groups change their diet from time to time, or digressions occur: adherents "sin," eating forbidden food. Nevertheless, some general conclusions can be drawn.

Regular vegetarians present no nutritional problems whatsoever. Exclusion of meat and fish from the diet in no way impairs health; vegetarians are able to obtain all the necessary substances from what they do eat. The "naturalistic" diet is, in the long run, more problematic. "Naturalists" must be very careful not to stick to a few food items, but should eat a rich and varied menu, including nuts, almonds, peanuts, etc., as well as many varieties of fruits—and, of course, grains such as wheat, oats, rice, etc. and dried legumes (beans, lentils, soy beans, peas, etc.). Only in this way can they avoid protein deficiency, although vitamin B_{12} deficiency may still occur. It so happens that "sinning" is often a saving grace.

The next questions are whether a "naturalistic" diet is superior, health wise, to a normal diet in any special way and whether it should be recommended. The diet is usually very poor in salt, with perhaps 1 to 2 grams daily, and very poor in saturated fat (some is present in peanuts and coconuts). It may be beneficial in cases of hypertension, in some cases of heart failure, in people with a high blood cholesterol, and in some cases of diabetes.

The same results can be obtained, however, by eating cooked foods containing meat, fish, etc., if they are properly planned. The idea that meat contains toxic materials, or that it is "not natural" to eat meat, is simply not true. Meat has been eaten by the human race since hunting began in prehistoric times. Meat and fish are easily and totally absorbed, and they contain amino acids and other elements that are essential to building body protein. As for their high fat content, one can chose to eat lean meat, liver, or kidneys, which are very low in fat. Excess visible fat can be trimmed and the meat grilled instead of fried. There is no evidence whatsoever that meat is unhealthful and therefore there is absolutely no need to renounce it.

The situation is quite similar with regard to cow's milk. This is the exclusive food on which many babies thrive, whose mothers do not breast-feed. It contains almost every substance needed by our bodies. There is no reason on earth why we should turn our backs on milk and milk products, though again the question of high fat content arises. But today one can buy low-fat milk (1 percent fat instead of 3 to 4 percent), "saving" 20 to 30 grams of fat per quart. There are also many low-fat cheeses and other milk products, such as yogurt.

Eggs are also rich in the best proteins and contain many vitamins. We can live without eggs, but why should we? They are a cheap source of good food, which can be prepared in many ways and served as a main dish. We do not have to eat several eggs daily, or put eggs into every recipe in cooking or baking, but there is absolutely no need to completely avoid eating eggs. (See pages 17–18.)

There appears to be no particular advantage in eating everything raw. Today, vegetables and fruits are more prominent in our diet than they were fifty years ago and a greater variety are now available. Many vegetables and fruits are eaten raw, supplying all the vitamin C needed, but cooking does not destroy more than about a quarter of the other vitamins, which are present in our food in more than sufficient quantities. Cooking does not in any way decrease the value of fruit or vegetable protein and carbohydrate, and, of course, many plants cannot reasonably be eaten raw at all. And let us not forget that the human race is known to have cooked food from the dawn of prehistoric time, which turns any attempt to label cooked food as "unnatural" into a grotesque.

Finally, the claims that certain vegetable or "naturalistic" diets have a healing effect on some diseases, prevent others, and prolong life have never been substantiated. Such claims rest primarily on anecdotal evidence. Humans are not mice, which can be kept indefinitely in cages so that long-term nutritional experiments may be made. This is especially true in the case of "naturalists" and other food-faddists, who often change their diets according to prevailing trends.

Summing up, one can say that while subsistence on a very varied "naturalistic" diet is possible, it is not recommended. Its advantages, such as low saturated fat and low salt intakes, can be achieved when necessary in a well-planned normal diet. The idea that meat is ordinarily toxic or contains toxic substances, or is not "natural" for us to eat, has absolutely no factual foundations. What is more, the anatomy and physiology of our digestive tract conform more to the meat-eating animal model than to that of the grazing species. No substantial evidence shows that a vegetarian or "naturalistic" diet has either a disease-preventing or life-prolonging effect.

"Scientific" Superstition

It has been related in the beginning of this chapter that the religions, and traditions, and folklore of many nations advise their people about what foods to eat in order to achieve certain aims, what foods to abstain from, and what foods should be sought for their healing effects. To folklore, tradition, and religious taboos, a new category has been added in the last few decades: pseudoscientific nutritional fads. It is nowadays easy to make people listen to dietary advice if a scientific explanation or theory goes along with it. Many fads have been introduced by popular books with a lot of fanfare—only to disappear from the scene a few years later. Eating protein and carbohydrates at different meals, so as not to mix them in the digestive process, is one fad that had absolutely no merit whatsoever but was nevertheless fervently defended by its adherents on "scientific grounds." Apple-vinegar and lecithin to combat obesity are also in this category. And now we have the "macrobiotic diet." What a beautiful scientific name!

Modern man's ear is tuned to novelty. We feel that a new diet *must* be better than the old ones, although experience should have taught us that this is not necessarily so. A more critical attitude is clearly indicated. It is the aim of this book to provide the reader with relevant information on what is known today, so as to strengthen his or her resistance to dietary superstitions—including pseudoscientific ones.

Conclusion

In an attempt to translate our present knowledge of nutrition into everyday practice, it seems reasonable to heed the significance of the recent revelations about fiber and legumes. It proves clearly that we do not yet know everything about the nutritional properties of all foods. Our mechanical classification of them into carbohydrates, fats, proteins, and vitamins and minerals—important as it may be—does not tell the whole story. And it is difficult to give totally sound advice before all the evidence is in. This is the fate of medicine: Physicians must interpret available knowledge in such a way as to cause the least possible harm and promote maximum usefulness.

The basic foods we eat, certainly the majority of them, have been eaten by mankind for many thousands of years. It stands to reason that foods containing extremely harmful substances would have been eliminated long ago. On the other, it is essential that we eat a great *variety* of foods. For several reasons. First, as stated above, we do not yet know all the nutritional values each food contains, so let us eat as many of them as possible. Second, the effects of *quantity* should be kept in mind: It is possible that certain foods may cause harm if ingested in large quantity. This point was made clear by what is now known about saturated fats; a small quantity of saturated fat is needed by the body and causes no evident harm, when the amount is greatly increased, as it has been in Western society in this century, it may well cause *disease.*

It has also become clear that our food should not be either too concentrated or too refined, such as are sugar, butter, chocolate, white bread, and fat cheeses, etc., or at least that we should consume such foods only in "reasonable" quantities. The question arises, of course, as to what is reasonable. We have seen that the average protein intake in our society has not increased, percent-wise, very much, and is about 16 percent of the calories we eat. The great deviation from the past seems to be our increase in fat consumption at the expense of carbohydrates, mainly grain. Meat, for example, is a rich source of fat. The high fat content is a property of domesticated farm animals; meat from wild animals, which was eaten by our hunting ancestors contained very little fat. In other words, it seems advisable to correct the aberrations that have developed rather recently in our affluent society. What we need are more carbohydrates, less fat, and less fiber-poor food.

To feed large urban populations, there is really no getting away from industrially processed food. But its fiber content and preparation should be kept as near as possible to the natural product. Food additives should be kept to an essential, well-tested minimum, as must pesticides.

How many meals should we have a day? One or two large ones, or several smaller ones? When should they be eaten? What is the proper sequence of dishes in a meal? Is hot or cold food better for us? Raw or cooked? Spiced or bland? These are some of the questions often asked of the medical profession!

Within countries of the affluent society, the answers to them vary greatly, depending on local customs, geography, climate, tradition, etc. And the answers do not seem to make much difference, certainly not to the extent that one way of eating can be pronounced significantly more healthful than the other.

It is worthwhile mentioning an experiment comparing the effect of three proper meals a day to eating exactly the same total amount of food divided into 17 equal "meals" (one each hour). The results seem to show that the latter is advantageous in some aspects, including blood cholesterol levels. However, much more data must be obtained before this finding can be accepted as definite.

Future Trends

The food industry is often accused of producing foods rich in sugar, fat, and salt, and this accusation is true to a large extent. And it is also true that home-cooked food is, in most families, also rich in these substances. According to U.S. law, the contents of a food product must be visibly marked on the package offered for sale, so that every consumer may know what he is buying if he cares to read this information. This information, however, is not always complete, often difficult to understand, and sometimes indirectly misleading. The laws covering food labeling must be overhauled and brought up to date.

Food producers are out to sell. They cater to consumers' whims and tastes. As long as consumers will pay higher prices for marbled steaks than for lean ones, producers will market fatty meat. If the demand for lean meat increases, its price will go up and the price of fatty meat will go down. Soon we will see more lean meat on the market. The same holds true for many other products, such as sausage and cheese; these can be produced with lower salt and fat content; but this will only happen in response to public demand; so let us not forget that food growing, processing, and production reflect the consumers' tastes and demand; it seems unjust to blame the industry because we like to buy and eat what is considered to be, onr the whole, unhealthful to us.

On the other hand, it seems that the food industry is rather conservative and does not exploit the many opportunities modern science could put at its disposal. Although consumers' eating habits are extremely difficult to change—a slow process and even a matter of generations—the food industry could change the *content* of various foods, instead of their taste and appearance, and thereby benefit consumers. With genetic engineering and other modern methods, an egg can be produced with very low cholesterol content and, what is more important, with less saturated and more unsaturated fat. (It is, of course, reasonable to believe that such eggs would fetch higher prices than regular ones.) With a little imagination, science could open new horizons for the food industry. If the public is interested, and willing to pay, we may in the not-too-distant future eat almost all we like and are used to, after undesirable substances have been removed, substituted for, or greatly reduced in quantity.

CHAPTER FIVE

Coffee — Innocent Despite Indictment

Where Does It Come From and How Is It Made?

Coffee is made from the roasted beans of the coffee plant, a small tree growing in tropical climates. The origin of the coffee tree is unknown, but it is assumed to have been growing wild in a southwestern Ethiopian province and called by the name of Kaffa. From here it was taken, around the end of the first millennium A.D., to southern Arabia and cultivated. It spread rather quickly through the Muslim world.

Coffee was introduced into Europe during the 16th and 17th centuries. Some claim this was done by the Turks, who advanced at the end of the 16th Century to the outskirts of Vienna. Others describe different routes of introduction. Be that as it may, during the 17th Century coffee became popular in many parts of Europe. Coffee houses flourished throughout the continent, and by the end of the century coffee was also sold in the British colonies in America.

At the beginning all coffee consumed in Europe originated in plantations in Arabia. With increasing demand, coffee growing spread to Ceylon and Indonesia. In the 18th Century coffee plants were introduced to South and Central America. The climate in these parts of the world seems to be most favorable to the coffee tree, especially at elevations of 1500 to 6000 feet. Most of the coffee production is now centered in this area—about half of the world production derives from Brazil alone. Significantly, the United States imports about half of the world's production of coffee.

After harvesting, the coffee beans undergo prolonged processes of washing, cleaning and drying. It is remarkable that there are no chemical tests for evaluating crops for quality. It can be done only by tasting—namely by applying the senses of taste and smell.

Roasting is the most important step in the processing of coffee. It imparts to the coffee its characteristic brown color and transforms the natural chemical constituents into new components that produce the desired aroma and taste. By adjusting temperature and duration of roasting, the flavor, degree of bitterness, and color are determined for the desired results. After roasting, coffee is ground and packed, or it is first packed and ground in the shop or at home.

Instant coffee, introduced during World War II, became quickly fashionable and widespread. The ease and rapidity of its preparation has made it increasingly popular. Instant coffee is prepared by liquid extraction of ground coffee.

In decaffeinated coffee, a large percentage of the caffeine is removed, without changing the taste too much. Originally, the process involved soaking a steaming extract of green coffee in a chlorinated organic solvent, which was later removed by washing out. Nowadays, most companies use only water. It is supposed to be marked on the jar or can, whether any chemicals were used in the process of decaffeination.

Caffeine and Other Ingredients

The major ingredient of coffee is caffeine. This substance is being used in various medications, though its indications and actions are not well defined. It is included in several anti-cold preparations and in various painkiller pills, especially for headache. It is questionable whether it has any remarkable pharmaceutical effect. Probably it is included in these preparations mainly for historical reasons. The effects of caffeine are to induce wakefulness and increase mental activity, to slightly enhance muscle work (by 2 to 3 percent), and to increase urine flow. On the other hand, in studies on athletes and in endurance tests, caffeine and coffee did not produce any appreciable improvement in performance.

The amount of caffeine varies greatly among the different coffee preparations. In a cup of filtered coffee there are about 120 milligrams of caffeine; in espresso, much more (up to two times the strength); in percolated coffee, about 80 milligrams; and in a cup of instant coffee, about 65 milligrams. A cup of tea contains about 60 milligrams of caffeine, almost as much as instant coffee. Caffeine is also present in cocoa, cola drinks, maté (a South American tea drink), and especially in chocolate. In a cup of decaffeinated coffee there are only about 2 to 3 milligrams of caffeine.

As the above figures prove, it is the mode of preparation that determines the amount of caffeine in a cup of coffee. The hot water, with which the ground coffee is treated, extracts a varying amount of the substance, according to the method used. The problem is how to extract the desirable flavoring substances with a minimum of bitter-tasting residues. It is well known that the temperature used must be below boiling, because boiling destroys the desirable aroma and flavoring. Furthermore, as the water temperature rises, the bitter components of coffee become increasingly soluble. Obviously, in addition to caffeine, other chemical substances are extracted from the beverage during its preparation.

These substances have not been thoroughly examined. They differ in composition and quantity among the various species of the coffee tree. The facility of their extraction depends not only on the mode of preparing the coffee, but also on the duration and temperature of roasting and the finesse of grinding.

The important role of the non-caffeine ingredients is emphasized by several effects of coffee, which are present also in decaffeinated coffee. First and foremost is the all-important aroma of coffee. And this is not due to caffeine! Furthermore, the effect of coffee on gastric secretions (see below) and on urine production is also not due to the caffeine, because it is present in decaffeinated coffee as well.

Coffee and Health

The major question is, of course, whether coffee endangers health or promotes any kind of disease. In the last few years alone, hundreds of medical publications have dealt with this question. It is characteristic of our times, but perhaps not surprising, that almost nobody has taken any interest in investigating tea, though it contains per cup almost the same amount of caffeine as instant coffee. But apparently a black beverage, which is drunk by many with great relish, and which many people crave, is suspect!

The possible relationship of coffee to almost any kind of disease has been exhaustively investigated. Many medical papers have been extensively reported and discussed in the daily press, in ways that often gave the impression that the public had good reason to be frightened. As so often happens, early, incomplete, and preliminary findings pointed to all kinds of negative reactions. Coffee was implicated as promoting a variety of cancers, such as cancer of the rectum, the bladder, the pancreas, and others. It was supposed to cause hypertension, all kinds of heart diseases—including myocardial infarction—a rise in blood cholesterol levels, increased birth defects in newborn babies, and much more.

However, additional *well-conceived and carefully executed studies failed to confirm any of the early findings.* Which only proves again that the "most recent findings" are not always the last word of absolute truth and wisdom. Let us never forget that next year there will be even more "recent findings"! It takes a lot of time and effort to find the errors and "bugs" in preliminary studies and to design an investigation that is able to uncover and understand the true state of affairs. Some of the early findings were truly bizarre, sounding almost like freaks of statistics: One study found that drinking five or more cups of coffee daily, *decreases* the chances of developing cancer of the colon by 40 percent!

Many doctors felt that coffee drinking promoted heart disease or harmed people with heart disease. Palpitations and disturbances in heart rhythm were thought to be most affected and were, accordingly, investigated with great care. Finally, no such association could be confirmed and coffee got a clean bill of health in this realm too.

Coffee and Cholesterol

For several years the medical world was embroiled in a dispute as to whether coffee drinking raises the blood cholesterol level. It all started with a Norwegian study in 1960, in which blood cholesterol levels were reported to rise progressively with increasing coffee ingestion. There followed a stream of studies in many countries, performed with different methods and techniques. The findings of the various studies differed to such an extent that one was inclined to ask oneself whether the investigated substance was really the same. Some found no effect, others a small effect, others found some effect in women but none in men, and vice versa. Recently, the Norwegian group reported, after studying some 12,000 people, that a significant (10 percent) increase in blood cholesterol levels was found only in people who consumed more than nine cups (!) of *boiled* coffee. This seems to be the preferred method of coffee preparation in Norway, and as far as is known is pretty much restricted to that country.

As always, it pays to listen to what the Framingham study has to say (see page 11). In a recent report released by the Framingham study staff on the effect of coffee intake on upward of 6000 people, including some 1000 with heart disease among them, *no increase in primary or secondary diseases of the heart were found!* Some changes in blood cholesterol were found only when more than nine cups were consumed daily.

The Effects of Coffee

So what are we left with? There are actually only two effects of any consequence: increase of gastric acid secretion and wakefulness. The first is not due to caffeine, as previously noted, but to some other substance extracted from coffee during cooking. In some people heartburn is produced after ingestion of coffee. The effect is more dramatic and harmful in people who suffer from peptic ulcer. Coffee is one of the three things forbidden to ulcer patients during an acute attack (the other two are cigarettes and alcohol).

As for wakefulness, this complaint is difficult to ascertain—and even more so to investigate. Some people claim that after drinking coffee in the evening they have difficulties falling asleep. It is rather astonishing that no such complaints are voiced after consumption of several cups of *tea* during the evening. This raises the—theoretical—question of whether wakefulness is not due to caffeine but to some other substance in the coffee bean. On the other hand, most—but not all—people who cannot fall asleep after drinking coffee have no such difficulty after ingestion of decaffeinated coffee.

Conclusions

If coffee prevents you from falling asleep, do not drink coffee in the evening, or try decaffeinated coffee. If you suffer from peptic ulcer disease, do not drink coffee during acute attacks and try to cut down on coffee between attacks.

For all the others there is absolutely no reason not to drink and not to *enjoy* their coffee. As so often in matters pertaining to health, it is not so much a question of yes or no, but a question of *how much*. The findings of all the medical trials reported in this chapter pertain to less than nine cups of coffee a day. A disproportionately high intake of coffee could perhaps cause some harm—just as very high intakes of many substances (even vitamins) could be harmful. Even on purely theoretical grounds it is not wise to exaggerate: Five cups a day is reasonable. If you must, drink two more cups—but do not exceed seven!

CHAPTER SIX

Alcohol—
Friend and Foe

Man's Best Friend

Alcohol as a beverage accompanies man from the dawn of his history; there is evidence that it was produced some 10,000 years ago, and doubtless some form of it was drunk even earlier. It was probably a serendipitous discovery: A fruit juice or other sugar-containing liquid fermented inadvertently; people tasted it, liked its effect; and spread it around the world.

There is hardly a grain or fruit grown on earth that is not used for the production of alcohol. Each country's sugar-containing plants serve as raw material: wheat, oats, barley, and potatoes in Europe, rice in the Far East, plums in the Balkans, cherries in Switzerland, cactus in Mexico, palm sap in India, grapes in all parts of the world where they can be grown, molasses, honey—all are used for making alcoholic drinks. There is no question as to alcohol's worldwide popularity. Alcohol has inspired artists in ancient as well as modern times. Poets have written of the "divine pleasures" of alcohol, devoting more poems to it than to any other subject except love and death. No celebration is complete, no party really starts going, and no good meal is perfect without alcohol.

Facts and Figures

The term "alcohol" refers to a group of organic substances with different characteristics, some of them very toxic. What we drink is actually ethyl alcohol, a simple alcohol containing two carbon atoms. Alcoholic beverages are basically of three kinds: (1) beer, usually brewed from malted barley, with various additives; (2) wine, the product of controlled fermentation, usually of grapes; and (3) spirits, the distilled and matured product of alcohol from grapes, barley, wheat, etc. Among the spirits, brandy is of grape origin. Rum is of molasses origin. And so on. Flavored spirits such as gin, aquavit, and absinthe are redistilled in the presence of flavoring agents. Liqueurs are flavored and sweetened spirits. All distilled alcoholic beverages are made up predominantly of alcohol and water. The characteristic flavor and aroma of each kind of spirit derives from very small quantities of organic compounds, called cogeners, which were carried over with the alcohol during the distillation process.

The alcohol content of a beverage is usually expressed as percentage of alcohol per total volume. It indicates the amount of milliliters (ml) of alcohol in 100 milliliters of beverage. Since alcohol is considerably lighter than water, its content "by volume" is actually about 20 percent higher than its content by weight. In other words, a wine of 10 percent alcohol by volume has only about 8 grams of alcohol per 100 milliliters. For spirits, alcohol content is expressed using the term "proof." Proof is about half of 1 percent alcohol by volume (1 proof = 0.5 percent). A spirit that is 80°, or 80 proof, contains 40 percent alcohol by volume, or about 33 grams of alcohol per 100 milliliters.

Beers contain 3 to 5 percent by volume, wines about 10 to 12 percent, and the strength of spirits is as indicated on the label of the bottle by proof: usually above 30 percent.

The Killer

The taste of good wine is exquisite and that of some superb vintages is so highly appreciated that one bottle can sell for thousands of dollars. Other drinks, such as champagne (sparkling wine), certain liqueurs, and very old cognac are a pleasure to our palate. But alcoholic beverages are not drunk simply for their taste—but for their effect.

That effect is typical of a drug. Small quantities have an elating and stimulating effect, while large quantities are intoxicating and eventually depressive. What happens in between is common knowledge. It is aptly and concisely summarized in an old Jewish saying: "In the first stage one feels like a lion, in the second stage one behaves like an ape, in the third stage one resembles a pig."

Beyond the first stage, alcohol's effect becomes destructive, immediately and in the long run. Drinking causes fights, irresponsible acts, absenteeism from work, car and industrial accidents—to mention just a few evils in a very long list. The long-range effect on a drinker's health is, mainly, but not exclusively, liver damage. Only a very small percentage of alcohol is excreted in the urine and in the exhaled air. More than 90 percent is metabolized in the liver. This process is called "detoxification." Small quantities of alcohol are easily handled by the liver, but there is a limit. Once drinking becomes an everyday affair and the quantities increase, liver damage ensues. The most dangerous form of alcoholic liver disease is cirrhosis, which in several Western countries is the third or fourth cause of death, after arteriosclerosis and cancer.

How Much Is Too Much?

Very few of the people who drink alcoholic beverages become addicts or chronic alcoholics. But these pose a serious problem so very familiar to Western societies that there is no need to elaborate on it. On the other hand, many people enjoy a few drinks and are not addicted. These people ought to know how much is harmful and when the limit is reached.

Those who occasionally drink too much may have a short-range problem, to be discussed below, but their liver is not endangered. On the other hand, those who drink regularly may have a potential liver problem, even if they are never totally drunk. The precise quantity of alcohol that causes cirrhosis depends on predisposing factors that are, as yet, not fully understood. This implies that there are great individual variations. It has, however, been established by research that daily intake over several years of more than 150 grams, or 5 ounces, of alcohol, will cause cirrhosis in close to 50 percent of drinkers. A French study has found that those who do not drink more than a one-liter bottle (about one quart) of wine daily will usually not be harmed. This corresponds to about 100 milliliters of alcohol by volume. For whiskey, the equivalent would be about 7 to 8 fluid ounces.

Many people who drink this much do not consider themselves alcoholics, nor would they be considered as such by others. A two-martini lunch, a highball after work, a predinner drink, a glass of wine at dinner, and maybe a beer or two while watching sports on television—or any similar combination—adds up to about 100 milliliters of alcohol. Those who drink regularly but are not addicts should figure out how much they drink daily. It is easily done, even without the help of a computer. But don't deceive yourself! To be on the safe side, the total amount should be kept *below* 100 milliliters for men, and lower for women—who are smaller than men and whose liver may be more susceptible. It goes without saying that during pregnancy no alcohol should be ingested, because of possible harm to the fetus.

Blood Levels and Drunkenness

When alcohol is drunk, these are the immediate effects: Absorption into the bloodstream is very rapid, since alcohol is one of the only three substances absorbed directly from the stomach (the other two are water and sugar). After a very short time, all of the alcohol drunk is in the bloodstream. After about half an hour to an hour, if one drinks on a full stomach, the blood level of alcohol is at its maximum. But the rate of elimination of alcohol from the blood is very slow indeed, amounting to a total of approximately 10 to 12 milliliters per hour.

The effects of alcohol correlate more or less with its level in the blood. People unused to drinking will show some mental impairment and disturbances of muscular coordination at an alcohol blood level of 0.05 percent, produced by drinking about 25 milliliters of alcohol. At blood levels of 0.1 percent (about 50 milliliters of alcohol), everybody, including regular drinkers, is unfit to drive a car. At 0.15 percent, or 75 milliliters of alcohol, everybody is obviously drunk. At 0.2 percent (100 milliliters), one is really in a bad state. From this level, it may take twelve hours and more to get the alcohol out of the system. When only a small amount is drunk, say 25 milliliters, the alcohol will be eliminated after three hours.

Here lies a remarkable difference between immediate and long-term effects of alcohol. As far as liver damage is concerned, it makes no difference whether one drinks 100 milliliters of alcohol at a time or whether it is distributed over the day. But it makes a big difference as far as drunkenness is concerned. Drunk within an hour or two, 100 milliliters will raise the blood level to about 0.2 percent and produce severe incapacitation for many hours. If the same quantity is divided into four periods of drinking about three to four hours apart, mental capacity, coordination, and inhibitions will not be impaired. This explains why some regular drinkers are surprised when their doctors tell them that they have cirrhosis of the liver—they never were actually drunk!

Calories

Those who are watching their weight should know that alcoholic beverages contain quite a lot of calories. One gram of alcohol contains about 7 calories. This is much more than in 1 gram of sugar or protein, almost as much as in 1 gram of fat. Practically, this means that one shot, or 1 ounce, of whiskey contains approximately 70 calories. A regular glass of wine contains about 150 calories if dry and up to 200 calories if sweet. A can or bottle of beer (a third of a quart) contains between 90 to 120 calories. Liqueurs have about 30 percent sugar added to the spirit, so one ounce may have 90 to 100 calories. So if you are on a diet, don't forget that alcoholic drinks do count!

Influence on Cholesterol and Heart Disease

Traditionally, doctors have prescribed a shot or two of cognac or whiskey daily to patients with arteriosclerotic heart disease. It dulls anginal pain, and may somehow widen the coronary arteries. Recent studies show; that the intake of 10 to 15 grams of alcohol daily lowers the cholesterol level in the blood. It appears that small quantities of alcohol have a good effect on arteriosclerotic patients, both immediately and in the long run.

Conclusions

This would be a good occasion to moralize. However, I will not do so, because I do not believe that addiction can be overcome by reasoning alone.

For those who are not addicted, small quantities of alcohol — 10 to 25 milliliters daily — are harmless. They may even be beneficial, except during pregnancy.

Those who do not drink habitually, but like to get a little high on special occasions, will also not be harmed permanently. Their problem is how to get home safely. If there is nobody to drive you home, do not think, "It won't happen to me" — take a cab. It is best to attend to this matter before the party starts and make appropriate arrangements.

Men who drink regularly should keep their alcohol intake below 100 milliliters daily (and women to less), so as to avoid liver disease.

Drinking 100 milliliters at a time will make everybody very drunk. Dividing the same quantity into three- or four-hour intervals between drinking will avoid drunkenness and not impair performance significantly.

You do not have to be a teetotaler to avoid being harmed by alcohol. Being familiar with quantities, understanding the characteristics and the effects of alcohol, and adhering to a few simple rules will permit you to enjoy it safely.

CHAPTER SEVEN

Tobacco's Smoke Signals

Where Did Tobacco Come From?

To most parts of the world, the use of tobacco is relatively new. It was adopted from the Indians of North America, and in the 16th Century was brought to Europe, where its use spread slowly during that and the following centuries. Tobacco leaves were processed and used in a wide variety of ways: for use in pipes and cigars, as snuff, as chewing tobacco, and finally, in the 19th Century, in the form of cigarettes. For all these products, except cigarettes, only tobacco leaves were used. For the production of cigarettes the tobacco was thinly cut and rolled in paper. This added a new dimension to smoking.

Cigarettes are the latest tobacco product. In the course of the 20th Century their use has increased, almost completely displacing chewing tobacco and snuff, and to a large extent even pipes and cigars. Today cigarettes account for most tobacco use. It is not quite clear why cigarettes gained such a popularity at the expense of all other uses of tobacco. Perhaps it was because cigarettes were much more convenient to use and carry wherever one went. Pipe smoking is more cumbersome and requires time for cleaning and filling. What's more, the aroma of pipe and cigar smoke is offensive to many people, and so both have become socially less acceptable. (Other reasons will be elaborated on later.)

Why Do People Smoke?

People smoke for the nicotine. Although the reason why people start smoking may be sociological or psychological, there is no doubt that eventually the exclusive reason for continuing to smoke is the will to experience the effects of nicotine. Time and again—from the beginning of this century—pharmacologists, chemists, and others have come up with nicotine-free cigarettes. Time and again it became clear that these cigarettes were not marketable. People have refused to smoke them. The oral gratification and other psychological benefits attributed to smoking are only negligible factors in the addiction to smoking.

The Effects of Nicotine

Nicotine produces, among its effects, behavioral changes, cardiovascular responses, and pulmonary reactions. Smoking is a gratifying experience. It is a reward that is highly anticipated. It produces, on the one hand, stimulation; on the other, a feeling of tranquillization and relaxation. Unlike many other drugs—e.g., alcohol or hashish—tobacco has no immediate negative side effects. It does not produce unpleasant changes of behavior that offend society. On the contrary, tobacco smoking can improve performance. This is the final reason why people smoke: It makes them feel better and it makes it easier for them to face difficult situations and perform better at work.

Smoking Behavior

Smoking behavior differs. Some people light an occasional cigarette, others smoke only after meals or at home after work, holding a cocktail in the other hand. Some smokers may drop the cigarette habit at will. But these are a small minority of smokers. Most smokers are actually addicted. They are unable to stop in spite of repeated health warnings, social pressure, and a full knowledge of the hazards involved. These are the smokers who would literally "walk a mile" for a cigarette.

Typically, people smoke a constant amount of cigarettes daily, except on special occasions, such as parties or conferences that drag into the night. The amount smoked daily may be fifteen cigarettes, a pack, or even two packs or more. Generally, every smoker keeps to his fixed dosage. And this implies a more or less constant interval between smokes. Someone smoking one pack a day will light a cigarette approximately every 45 minutes. If unable to do so, he or she will feel the urge anyway, and touch his pockets as if to make sure the cigarettes are still there. When cigarettes with a lower nicotine content are substituted for a smoker's regular brand, the interval between cigarettes will shorten and the total number smoked will increase.

The *rate* of smoking is probably regulated by the blood level of nicotine or by the rate of its excretion from the blood and urine. This dose-related addiction accounts for the fact that heavy smokers usually cannot cut down on their smoking. A decision to smoke one pack daily instead of two is usually not sustained for any length of time. For these smokers it may be even easier to stop smoking completely than to reduce the number of cigarettes smoked! Moreover, those who stop for some time— even for years—and start again with just a few cigarettes a day, will shortly find themselves smoking at the previous rate, no more and no less.

The Detrimental Long-Term
Effect on Health

The effect of cigarette smoking on health is clearly established by statistics covering millions of people, amassed over the last three decades. The first smoking-related diseases to be identified were chronic bronchitis and chronic lung disease, which almost totally impede the vital gas exchange between lungs and blood. The clear-cut, dose-dependent relationship between lung cancer and cigarettes followed. Finally, it has been proven that the heart is also severely affected by cigarette smoking. The incidence of heart attacks in cigarette smokers is much higher than in nonsmokers, reaching alarming proportions in heavy smokers. Heavy cigarette smoking is recognized today as the number one "risk factor" for heart attacks.

The effect of smoking on these and other cigarette-related diseases is "dose" dependent. Below five cigarettes daily there is very little danger. With above ten, morbidity and mortality increase sharply. A pack is dangerous, and anything above a pack must be considered extremely dangerous.

And Other Tobacco Products?

Statistics on all other tobacco products present a different picture. Cigar and pipe smoking are far less dangerous than cigarette smoking. Up to nine pipes a day and up to five cigars daily appear to cause only a small increase in smoking-associated diseases. Even higher doses cause relatively little harm. The reason may be that less tar and less carbon monoxide (CO) are inhaled. Statistically significant data for snuffing and chewing tobacco are nowadays extremely difficult to come by. Judging from what figures are available, it seems that they too are relatively harmless, as far as lung and heart disease are concerned, but local damage, even cancer of the gums and mouth, may be produced.

Obviously, cigarettes are the most hazardous species of the

"tobacco family." This seems to indicate that the harmful substance is not nicotine. It may be tar, the smoke of the burning paper, or perhaps other substances not yet identified or tested. The problem may be the organ to which the smoke is directed, lung tissue being very susceptible to disease. Most cigar or pipe smokers do not inhale, or inhale very little. The nicotine and the other substances are absorbed from the oral and inner nasal surfaces. The same is true of snuff and chewing tobacco. Nicotine from cigarette smoke, on the other hand, is absorbed into the lungs. Absorption from the lungs is quicker and therefore more satisfying. Every cigarette smoker knows that the first inhalation produces immediate effect. This is, most probably, one of the major reasons for the popularity of cigarettes.

Who Smokes When

All that has been said so far is scientifically established and is taught to doctors, nurses, and other medical personnel. It is also well known to the general public. In spite of it, 40 to 60 percent of the male population in many countries are still smoking cigarettes. Perhaps a *remote* danger is not an effective deterrent. This is apparent from the smoking pattern in the United States, here, the onset of smoking is now at a much earlier age than previously. Smoking among teenagers is common, and even preteens are not exempt. Perhaps parents have less influence than they used to have. Perhaps, being smokers themselves, many parents cannot reason with their children. And some may feel—rightly or wrongly—that cigarettes are preferable to marijuana.

Women have also taken up smoking in the last five or six decades. Until World War II, smoking was primarily a male affair, but today the percentage of women smokers approaches that of men. On the other hand, the percentage of adult men who indulge in smoking has decreased markedly. It seems that the older a man gets—the closer to the day of reckoning—the more he is inclined to heed the warnings.

The new demographic distribution of cigarette smoking

accounts for the fact that the total number of smokers and the total number of cigarettes produced in the U.S. have decreased in the last two decades, though at a rate, which up to very recently did not seem sufficiently responsive to the relentless, well-publicized anti-smoking campaigns.

How About Stopping?

Some people are fatalistic. So many things may happen, life is full of dangers, so let us at least enjoy cigarettes. Others may believe that it is not going to happen to them. Like a certain cab driver who was chain-smoking: A fare told him, "Don't you know it's dangerous?" "Yes, my grandfather was a heavy smoker and he died of lung cancer." "You see!" "When he was ninety-five years old." But most adult smokers must have contemplated stopping at one time or another. Many have probably tried, perhaps several times, without success.

People who smoke only occasionally, or less than ten cigarettes daily, can usually quit smoking quite easily, or limit themselves to three to five cigarettes daily. These people are, however, only a small percentage of the smokers and they are not the problem.

For the others, quitting poses a problem—but not an insurmountable one. For most people it is futile to "stop gradually" by slowly cutting down daily consumption, although sometimes this may work. The halt must be made suddenly and completely! You extinguish the cigarette you are smoking and—never again! In the first two to three weeks there will be a strong craving for cigarettes, which subsides only gradually. During the first, and sometimes even during the second, month, a former smoker may experience depression and irritability. He or she may be nervous, short-tempered, and a temporary nuisance to family and fellow workers. Or weight may be gained. People don't lose weight when they start smoking, but they do gain, at least temporarily, after stopping. Family members can be helpful. If they support your effort and count the days with you, they will make it more difficult for you to relapse. If you don't smoke for one full month, you have a good prospect for success. Needless to say, never smoke a cigarette again. Not even a single one. It may be your undoing!

Some individuals are helped by hypnosis, others by indirect suggestion, such as acupuncture, or by other means and devices. Often it helps if you quit together with your spouse or a friend. This way, you can exchange experiences.

To quit smoking is not easy. If it were, practically every smoker would do so. Many have failed because they did not know what to expect, and found it more difficult than they imagined. If you have failed before, you may succeed if you try a second or third time, if you are ready for a difficult month or two. Millions have succeeded, among them some very heavy smokers.

What If I Cannot Stop?

Nevertheless, some people are not capable of kicking the habit for any length of time. In these hard-core cases, prodding and warning are of no avail. They are convinced of the danger, but find it beyond their power to stop. They should be encouraged to make an effort to switch to pipe or cigar smoking. Many who have tried and failed in their effort to stop cigarette smoking have managed to switch to a pipe or to cigars. The "exchange" is not an ideal solution, but it is still less dangerous than continuing to smoke cigarettes.

And do not forget that nicotine-containing chewing gum is commercially available. It provides less immediate gratification, but it still gives you a relatively less harmful nicotine—without the ill effects of cigarette smoke.

CHAPTER EIGHT

Your Weight
and Your Health

What Is Obesity?

Obesity means excess of fat tissue. Fat tissue is an essential component of the body, concentrated mainly subcutaneously (below the skin) where it is deposited in varying quantities in every normal human being. Fat tissue can also be found in many other organs, most pronounced in the abdomen in the coverings of the bowels. Men tend to collect excess fat mostly in the abdomen, and women in the breasts, thighs, and buttocks. Horrifying pictures of people emaciated from hunger, which has not yet disappeared from the world, show bodies with an almost complete absence of fat tissue. This demonstrates in the extreme where fat tissue is normally accumulated and its dramatic effect on our appearance.

Fat is the only means the human body has to store energy, since very few carbohydrates and no proteins at all are stored.

The body uses this stored fat according to its needs, converting it into fuel to activate normal metabolic processes which require energy.

Generally, the degree of obesity can be determined simply by one's weight. But being overweight does not automatically indicate obesity. Once while examining a group of young men about to be drafted into the army, I was handed a chart of an eighteen-year-old boy who was undressing in the adjoining room. I read that he was 5 feet 5 inches tall, and weighed 220 pounds! On my way to the other room to examine him, I thought that the chances of making a soldier out of this fat little fellow were slight indeed. When I saw him, I could not suppress my laughter. He was a weight lifter, with extraordinarily developed muscles and, if anything, less fat tissue than an average boy his age. Here was an extreme case of being overweight with no obesity!

Another condition that causes an increase of weight that is unrelated to obesity is water retention which can be due to a variety of diseases.

Usually, as one gets older muscles atrophy and more fat is accumulated by the body. This was best explained by a well known World War II general's wife. She said, when asked about her husband's weight; "His weight is the same as it was at West Point, only now it is in different places."

There are several elaborate methods to determine the true fat content of the body, such as weighing someone under water to calculate a person's specific gravity. (Fat tissue is lighter than muscular tissue. It follows that the lower a person's specific gravity, the higher the percentage of fat. A person immersed under water displaces an amount of water equal to his body's volume. Knowledge of volume and weight permits calculating specific gravity.) These methods are only used in scientific research. Some doctors measure the thickness of the skin folds of the arm, chest, and other parts of the body to determine one's fat content as it is relates to one's weight. Usually, however, there is no need for these procedures. In normally built people their weight is a sufficient indication of the body's fat content.

One's Normal Weight

To the simple question, "How much should I weigh?", there is just no simple answer, but there is an answer to "How much is too much?" It has never been scientifically determined what the optimal weight for each individual should be. It would be very difficult to determine the criteria on which such an analysis should be based. What is available are charts published by the Metropolitan Life Insurance Co. starting from the end of the 19th Century, relating optimal weight to height. This is based on averages they have computed from their healthy insured population. What this chart actually conveys is not how much one should weigh, but rather the weight of the average healthy American. Their latest figures, released in the early 1980s, allow a few pounds more than their previous set of figures. Does this mean that to be healthy you should now weigh more than before? Of course not. It only denotes that the average healthy person in the U.S. is now a few pounds heavier than the healthy person of the previous generation.

These charts are reproduced in textbooks for physicians, dietitians, etc. and in many publications read by the general public. They are accepted as "Normal Weight," and rightly so, since for now this is the best science has to offer us.

Usually these charts contain three columns for every weight: small, medium, and large "frame." The word "frame" is not defined. It does not stand for skeletal frame, whatever this may mean, nor does it indicate people who have thick bones or well developed muscles. No such correlative study has ever been performed. It stands simply for those who are 10 percent below average ("small frame") and those who are 10 percent above ("large frame"). Many of my obese patients, who looked broad-shouldered and very "large frame," became definitely "small frame" after losing weight.

Being obese carries with it the risk of contracting many diseases. This risk increases with the degree of obesity. What might be termed "medical obesity," meaning obesity which presents medical problems, begins at about 5 percent to 10 percent above the upper limit of the "large frame" category.

But as we shall see, there are other aspects to this problem beside the medical ones.

Obesity and Society

In poor societies obesity is actually looked upon as indicating health and affluence. In the Bible the literal translation of the word meaning "healthy" also has the connotation of fat. This is understandable because fat tissue (representing the body's reserve of energy) was highly desirable during the biblical times of frequent famines and numerous dangerous parasitic or bacterial diseases. It is no small wonder that in primitive tribes and in countries where it is customary to pay for brides, the fatter ones have the greater perceived value and fetch the highest prices.

This mentality changes completely with the rise of living standards. In today's affluent societies the admired body-image (or form) is trim and lean, with slight variations in countries with somewhat lower standards of living. A woman considered to be on the fat side in New York, will still be whistled at admiringly in Sicily, not to mention the commotion she may cause in a Near-Eastern bazaar.

A study performed on the New York City population found that women from the higher echelons of society were leaner than those from the lower ones. Another study showed that third-generation American women were leaner than women of the second generation of the same ethnic origin and age who were again leaner than those who were their first-generation relatives.

All this clearly proves that our views as to who is obese and who is not are based more on social norms than anything else. We do not really need charts, averages, norms, and all kinds of calculations of height, sex, and age. All we need to do is look in the mirror. Looking at people on the street, or any other place one meets people, we know immediately who is obese, who is just a little fat, who is normal, and who is too thin.

This implies that in addition to what can be termed

"medical obesity," meaning obesity which is medically undesirable, there is also "social obesity." Social obesity is present when one's fat tissue exceeds what is compatible with the society's social norm, and it is totally in the eyes of the beholder. Social obesity in Western society today starts at a lower weight level than medical obesity. This means that both sexes, and especially women, will be considered obese by society at a degree of weight which is not yet medically dangerous.

B. W. Roper, the former president of the American Association for Public Opinion Research, told this interesting story about being overweight: ". . . In the course of a survey, respondents were asked their height and weight. They were also asked their opinion about their fatness or slimness. . . . When the results were tabulated and compared to the Metropolitan Life Insurance company's height and weight charts, there was a consistent discrepancy between what responders thought of their weight and how the Metropolitan height and weight charts classified people. Those who regarded themselves as substantially overweight were only slightly overweight according to the Metropolitan charts. Those who regarded themselves as a little overweight were just right according to the Metropolitan charts, etc.

"Three or four years later Metropolitan revised its height and weight charts. When we looked again at this survey we found that respondents' estimates now conformed to the revised Metropolitan judgments. Thus, an opinion poll provided more accurate measurement of overweight than the experts did—until the experts revised their judgment." *

Types of Obesity

Many obese people believe that their condition is caused by some kind of disease, like "hormonal imbalance" or the like. Medical examinations only very rarely reveal an associated disease. Being overweight with edema of the lower extremities

---

*From *The Annals of the American Academy of Political and Social Science* (March 1984).

or accumulation of fluid in the abdomen may be a sign of liver, kidney, or heart disease, but it is actually due to retention of water and not to the accumulation of fat tissue and has nothing to do with obesity.

In a small minority of people, perhaps 5 in 1000 cases or less, one of two different hormonal obesity diseases may be found. One is the excessive secretion of adrenal hormones, known as Cushing's disease, which is extremely rare. It presents many severe symptoms including a special type of obesity affecting one's trunk and neck, producing a round face ("moon face"), and relatively thin extremities. The other disease is inadequate functioning of the thyroid gland, known as hypothyroidism. In this disease there might be some increase in fat tissue. Most of the weight gained, however, is due to a gelatinous substance deposited under the skin and in other organs. It can be eliminated through thyroid replacement therapy. In both diseases weight gain is not the major symptom, and the effects of the other symptoms are more pronounced and troublesome. Under medical examination these conditions can readily be distinguished from obesity.

Another rare form of obesity is the so-called morbid or monstrous obesity. People with the affliction weigh two or three times what is normal and they usually continue gaining weight. Their pictures occasionally appear in the newspapers and some of them are even mentioned in *The Guinness Book of World Records.* This is a disease which is in many cases familial, the cause of which has not yet been figured out. It is probably due to changes in one or more of the vital centers in the brain, which are directly or indirectly concerned with the regulation of food intake.

The remaining 99 percent or so of obese people are just plain obese. No disease or pathological factor can be diagnosed, even after the most extended and probing examination. In other words, this is simple or constitutional obesity. More women than men are overweight. Records show that in some treatment series women outnumber men four to one, but this is not the real ratio, since women are more sensitive about their appearance and also look more readily for medical help.

The medical histories of people with simple obesity problems are usually not significant. The parents may or may not be obese, but in most cases at least one of them is. Modern research, including identical twin studies, puts more and more emphasis on genetic factors. Obese people often report that they were chubby babies. They were overweight in grade school, and at college and into their adult lives. Some women gained additional weight during pregnancy, and were unable to lose it afterwards. Some obese people were normal as children, or perhaps even underweight, and their obesity started after an illness. And sometimes it manifested itself between the ages of six to ten years or in girls with the onset of puberty.

Most overweight people have tried desperately to lose weight. They have dieted at various points of their lives, often successfully. Some have reached more or less normal weight, once or even several times, but sooner or later they gained it all back again. Not infrequently, transient obesity appears in girls in their teens who were of normal weight until this time. Sudden weight gain may happen in high school or college, and is sometimes associated with temporary arrest of regles. The good news is that after two or three years, most overweight girls go on serious diets, usually without consulting a doctor or a dietitian, lose their excess weight, and stay within or close to the socially accepted norm.

The distribution in our bodies of excess fat follows the same patterns as normal fat-tissue. Usually the distribution of fat in the subcutaneous tissue is more or less even all over the body and our trunk, limbs, and face are all endowed with some excess fat. In addition there are sexual differences. In men, fat is most often found in the abdomen, beginning with the appearance of the so called "spare tire" around the middle of the body. In women, excess fat usually settles in the thighs, buttocks, lower part of the abdomen, and the breasts. In some women the upper part of their body is inexplicably more or less normal, while fat is accumulated in the lower part of their body. This distribution is genetically determined. When losing weight, fat tissue decreases everywhere. Quite often, especially in this type of obesity, not as much is lost as would be desirable in places that are most heavily padded.

The Causes of Obesity

The causes of obesity are unknown. Everybody knows, of course, that it is directly related to the amount of food eaten. This can easily be proven, since by decreasing the amount of food intake one loses weight. How much we eat is determined by appetite. But hunger and appetite are not the same. They are not even different degrees of the same phenomenon. Hunger is an unpleasant sensation, a reaction to starvation. The lining of the stomach grows pale and does not secrete digestive juices. From time to time the stomach contracts, and "pangs" are experienced. Appetite is quite another matter. The gastric mucosa is red and actively secreting. It is a pleasant feeling, completely unrelated to hunger, and may even be present after a full meal when we see or smell a dish we like.

Appetite is a complex sensation. The appetite center or centers in the brain are influenced by much feedback. Positive feedback is caused by agreeable smells and negative feedback by repulsive ones. Other influences are the degree of fullness of the stomach, the amount of food recently ingested, the quantity and composition of food, dizziness, nausea, as well as blood levels of various biochemical substances related and unrelated to food, and many others.

Deviations from normal body weight are often attributed to a disturbance of appetite. But why does an obese person eat more than is needed to sustain normal weight? To answer this and other specific questions about weight we have to rely mainly on assumption and hypothesis. Why do very lean people eat less? Which factors have a dominant influence on the appetite center? Are these factors biochemical, hormonal, physical, or psychological? Though no definite answer can be given at present, we can deduce some answers from known facts and observations which may serve as circumstantial evidence.

Maintaining Constant Body Weight

Almost all healthy adults of normal weight maintain a more or less constant weight throughout their adult lives. This is true for both sexes, though it is more easily observed in men. In women, pregnancies, lactation and some water retention preceding menstruation may obscure the picture, but not basically change it.

The average quantity of food that we consume daily is on the order of 2500 calories. This amounts to about 1,000,000 calories a year. To produce one pound of fat tissue some 3200 calories are required. Assuming a constant weight over thirty years, the gain or loss of five pounds would give the following result: of 30,000,000 calories eaten, 32,000 calories are the combined deviation of ten pounds (five up and five down). This indicates a precision of about one tenth of one percent (0.1%). This is an extraordinary, almost astonishing precision, as biological feedback mechanisms go. It really means that the body regulates our food intake almost exclusively through the appetite, with extreme accuracy. It, thereby, keeps fat tissue within the individual's predetermined very narrow limits. In other words, the amount of fat tissue in every individual is kept constant by an as yet unknown feedback mechanism, just as other physiological mechanisms keep body temperature, content of salts, and other biochemical substances constant. It follows that certain physiological mechanisms have a clear "body image" (unrelated to what psychologists call by the same name) to which the body adheres closely.

The existence of such a regulatory mechanism is evident in many examples found in our everyday lives. For example: A young man contracts an infectious disease. In the course of the disease he develops a high fever and he loses seven pounds. After recovering he is weak and his doctor sends him to spend a week or two in a convalescent home. The institution serves excellent food five times a day. The young man will rapidly regain the seven pounds that have been lost and will most probably stop gaining weight at this point. Should he come home with an excess pound or two he will soon shed them and revert to his normal, pre-sickness weight.

In another example: A student leading a sedentary life, takes on a summer job which requires physical exertion. He spends about fifty percent more energy (calories) at this job than at college. He may initially lose some weight, but after two to three weeks he will start gaining, until his normal, pre-working weight is attained. This proves that appetite adjusts rather quickly to changes in energy expenditure. When giving up smoking people may gain a few pounds, but they will usually shed them after a few months. Additional examples of these phenomena could easily be provided, but since everyone has had the occasion to observe some in their life, we need not belabor the point.

What about fat people? Do they also have an appetite regulating mechanism which always keeps their weight constant? Yes, it seems so. It is the same with most fat people, except, of course, those who suffer from morbid or monstrous obesity. The difference is that the appetite regulating mechanism of the obese is set at a higher level. Years ago I treated a series of thirty patients who lost 22 to 143 pounds on dietary treatment. Fourteen years later twenty-seven of them were located and reexamined. All but three were back within five pounds of their pre-dietary weight of fourteen years before. It was not surprising that they had regained their original weight. This has been described in medical literature before. What did surprise me was that they had actually returned to their constant weight without adding more. fat over the period of fourteen years.

The same is true of very lean people. They too maintain their below-normal weight. If there is anything more difficult than keeping a fat person's weight down for any length of time, it is trying to make thin people gain weight.

Evidently fat people, like normal and thin ones, keep their body weight constant throughout most of their adult lives. This is obscured by episodes of dieting, by pregnancies, etc. but basically it always holds true.

Mrs. R. is a good example. She first came to see me when she was thirty years old. She was 5'4" tall and weighed 185 pounds, about forty percent overweight. She explained that this had been her weight since she was an adult. She lost some 35 pounds by dieting and was happy to be only ten percent overweight. After three years she came to my office again, saying that she kept her post-diet weight for six months and than started slowly gaining. After another twelve months she was 185 pounds again and it took her one and a half years before deciding to try dieting again. This was repeated over the years another two times, in exactly the same pattern and weight fluctuations till I told her that now she knew as much or more about losing weight as I did. I lost sight of her, but she is probably still at it.

Psychology and Obesity

We have seen that the amount of fat tissue in our body is kept constant by physiological mechanisms. If this is so, then there is absolutely no basis to the claims that obesity is caused by psychological factors. There is no proof whatever that fat people overeat "in order to compensate for difficulties in life" or that they are "hopelessly addicted to food" or that if they would only apply more "willpower" everything would be all right, including their figure. Obese people have been made to undergo psychiatric treatment, both singly and in group therapy situations and the resulting benefits are virtually nonexistent. This is another indication that the causative factor is not a psychological one. Of course, fat people can have psychological problems, sometimes serious ones. This is largely due to society's negative attitude to obesity, beginning in the school years and continuing with the constant prodding and moralizing to which they are subjected by family and friends. It is true that in times of stress fat people eat more than usual and tend to gain weight, just as thin people lose weight in such times. This is caused by people relaxing a certain measure of their self-control that is normally exercised. In no way does this imply that the causative factor of obesity is found in the realm of psychology. Accusing fat people of "weakness of character" is totally unjustified and adds to the troubles of people who already suffer too much because their figures are perceived to be unesthetic in the eyes of today's society.

Fat Babies

Since many fat babies grow up to be obese adults, the question of *why* some babies are fat is relevant in determining the cause of obesity. Theoretically, the possibility that this may be caused by psychological factors cannot be completely eliminated. However it is very unlikely. Moreover, no evidence has ever been presented that fat babies are unhappier than other babies or have a "deprived babyhood." Pediatricians used to blame mothers for overfeeding their babies, by giving them more or calorie-richer food. Perhaps some mothers in the past had such intentions, but given modern society's attitude towards obesity, it is highly improbable that today's mothers want fat babies.

Who actually determines how much a baby eats? Experience, shared by most parents, indicates that the baby does. If parents are instructed by the pediatrician to feed every four hours, but after three hours the baby screams its head off because it is hungry, what should the parents do? They naturally feed the baby after three hours! Other babies may refuse to finish their bottle, and nothing helps. If they are forced to eat, they vomit. There seems to be little doubt that in this matter the baby is stronger than its parents and their doctors. The baby eats according to its own appetite-regulating mechanism.

Do Fat People Overeat?

The questions are often asked: Do fat people eat a lot? Do they overeat? Obtaining a reliable nutritional history is difficult, even in the best of cases, when the patient cooperates fully. It is almost impossible to determine the true nutritional history from people who try to convince themselves and others that they do not eat too much. Who remembers what he had for lunch the day before yesterday? How much butter did he spread on his bread? How many slices of bread did he eat? And that cake at the office party, how much of it did he eat? What was it made of, how much fat was in it, and what other ingredients did it contain? It gets even more difficult if one eats in a restaurant. After all who knows what the cook has actually put into a dish? And how many beers and shots of whiskey did the person being interviewed drink at his friend's birthday party? What about the peanuts? etc., etc.

It is very hard to answer these questions correctly. To know what others really eat, at mealtimes and between meals, is impossible. Nevertheless, it is quite obvious that most fat people, when not temporarily on a reducing diet, eat much and with gusto. I have seen a thin person forget a meal when he was busy or preoccupied, but never a fat person. They may forgo a meal consciously, but they will never forget that it is mealtime.

But, the fact that they usually eat relatively large quantities does not mean that they overeat. If everyone eats what is required to sustain his or her weight, then the term "overeating" is not applicable. The facts and observations detailed so far describe what is common to all people, whether normal, fat, or thin. The common denominator of all people is that everyone eats according to his own appetite-regulating mechanism. The difference is that in each person the regulator is set on a different amount of fat tissue: that is, at a different weight. Those whose triggering point is within the socially accepted norm are lucky. Those whose triggering points are too high have a lifelong struggle with diets. They will often try, with pathetic continuing failure, to bring their weight down to fit the acceptable social norm.

Principles of Treatment

By now it should be clear that losing excess fat or avoiding its formation is neither simple nor easy. *Obesity is a chronic, lifelong condition.* This is the basic fact that must be taken into consideration when attempting to fight it. To regard it as a passing condition is absolutely ridiculous, just as is telling your friends "I have lost two pounds the past ten days." Almost every obese person, with very few exceptions, has lost weight by dieting. Some have taken off weight so many times, that when adding up all the pounds lost in the course of their lives the total easily exceeds their weight. Nevertheless, they still remain fat.

The results of reducing diets are disappointing. Most

studies report that within a year about 90 percent of those who started treatment are back at their pre-diet weight. It makes little difference what kind of diet is chosen, the long-term results seem to be the same. Whether it is a regular reducing diet, focusing on normal food items, a liquid diet, a special diet such as not mixing carbohydrates with proteins, just fasting—it is always the same: After a year or two about 90 percent are right back where they started. The same goes for the so-called "behavioral" therapy, where people are taught to change their eating habits. Some doctors have gone so far as to resort to wiring patients' teeth, with their complete encouragement. This is so cruel a procedure that had it been done to animals, the ASPCA would certainly have intervened. Even this drastic procedure did not keep the weight off for more than the short run.

It is beyond reasonable doubt that the problem is not how to lose weight but how to keep to the post-diet weight!

It is amusing to read every few months about some new miracle diet that is on the market. It is pathetic how many obese people follow it religiously for a few weeks or months, with the same results as before. There is no miracle diet, and there never will be. To be effective, a diet must contain less food, i.e., fewer calories, than is necessary to satisfy the overweight person's appetite-regulating triggerpoint. Otherwise the weight cannot come off in the first place. This is very unpleasant and hard to endure, no matter what the diet is composed of and no matter what special features or trimmings it contains. If there *were* an easy why to maintain the post-diet weight level and not gain in back again, no diets at all would be needed. Every fat person would merely restrict his food intake for as long as necessary to achieve a normal weight. When it comes to losing weight, most and probably all obese people have proven time and again they can do so. Keeping it off is another story.

A Few Don'ts

Don't take weight-reducing drugs. None of the drugs available at present will help to reduce weight for any length of time.

Many of them are ineffective and others have severe and sometimes dangerous side-effects. The long-range results with drugs are no better than results without them, and they are often worse.

Don't Fast. Radical food deprivation can compromise your health and even cause death. Many fatal cases are on record. The long-term results of fasting are no better than those of dieting. Whatever you do, don't yield to the temptation to take all the weight off at once.

Don't Reach for Wonder Drugs and Miracle Cures. Losing weight through dieting is not easy, and causes much suffering. Nobody has discovered a painless way to lose weight. There are so-called reducing establishments, which will put you into special impermeable suits or layers of wax to make you perspire. After an hour or two you go home happy, lighter by two three pounds. Unfortunately, what you have lost is sweat, meaning water, and not one gram of fat. Other establishments will inject you with various hormones telling you that dieting will now be painless. However, it has been proven by controlled experiments that there are no known hormones that facilitate dieting. Nor can existing drugs make your fat tissue dissolve or melt away. So far a drug which will make excess fat just disappear the easy way has not been discovered. Should such a drug or cure become available, you can be sure that the whole world will know about it in no time. There is no reason to believe the multitudes of weight-reducing advertisements that push weight reducing wonders that simply do not exist. You won't lose the weight nor is it good for your morale to follow every fad and discover that you have been fooled again. Whether the creators of new diets have good intentions or not makes little difference.

Don't Restrict Salt Intake in Order to Lose Weight. Some people with heart, kidney, or liver disease have a problem with water accumulation in their bodies. This causes unusual weight gain, with swelling of the lower extremities and sometimes of the abdomen. This type of weight gain is easily distinguished from obesity. Treatments for this type of weight gain include salt restrictions or diuretics, among others. Since water retention causes weight gain, the mistaken idea has somehow developed, that salt restriction or even diuretics may help to lose fat. This is utterly untrue. Salt restriction in no way affects obesity, nor does it help to lose weight. Diuretics taken without medical supervision may be dangerous. There are cases on record of people having been seriously harmed by diuretics taken in the fond hope that this will be their path to slimness.

Don't make it the major topic of conversation with family and friends. If you are on a diet there is no reason to hide it from your friends, and your family will know about it anyway. If you succeed in losing any appreciable amount of weight, everybody will notice it. On the other hand, it is often helpful to discuss your diet with people who have the same problem, and many find "Weight Watchers" or similar organizations helpful. This usually involves meeting weekly with other people who are trying to lose weight, exchanging experiences, and encouraging each other. But this does not mean that you have to let your family and friends in on all the details of your diet, on every pound you lost or did not lose. Though it may be entertaining for a while, it will finally begin boring them. Surely there are more interesting topics of conversation—so don't overdo it.

How to Go About It?

You must know that losing weight is only the first step, and that you are facing a chronic problem that will be with you all your life. You must know that in order to have any lasting effect the diet you have decided on is only the beginning of a diet that will be ongoing for many, many years, perhaps for the rest of your life. It will not have to be as rigorous as the initial weight-loss period, but you will never be able to eat all you want. In other words, once a diet—always a diet, day in and day out, 24 hours a day. If you are not prepared for this type of commitment there is no use trying. All you will achieve will be temporary weight loss while rapidly regaining it back. You will be paying a high price in personal deprivation and most of the time you will be on the obese side. It is essential therefore, that you approach dieting with the utmost of seriousness and commitment so it does not turn into a futile, lifelong, frustrating effort.

Basically there are two kinds of diets: *weight-loss diets* and *maintenance diets.* Those that lose weight involve considerably fewer calories than those that maintain it, but since the weight-losing aspect of the diet is generally in effect for only short periods of time it is easier to bear than the lifelong requirements of the maintaining diet. The crucial commitment must be to the maintenance diet, which you have to adhere to forever if you want to succeed. Before starting to reduce, you should decide exactly how much you want to lose. The target must be clear and predetermined if you really want to achieve it.

A good idea would be to first lose fifteen pounds. This can be achieved in five to six weeks on a reducing diet involving normal food (to be discussed later). Start the diet at home, in your usual surroundings, proceeding with your work, be it at home or in an office, a factory, or a store. There is no point in going to a spa or a "fat farm" because all you will learn is that you can diet effectively at special institutions, but not at your home. So what is the big accomplishment? If you cannot succeed at home, with your family, work, and other normal obligations, your success will certainly be short-lived.

The next step is to keep your new weight level for six months without gaining! This can be achieved with the help of a maintenance diet (to be discussed later).

Having succeeded so far, you may again start on a weight-loss diet, to cut another fifteen pounds. Then back again to the maintenance diet for another six months. This can be repeated until you reach your predetermined weight. If you are ten percent to twenty percent overweight, you can aim for what your normal weight should be. If you are more than twenty percent overweight, your normal weight plus ten percent is a more realistic target to aim for, and much easier to sustain.

The Weight-Loss Diet

This must be a low-calorie diet to be effective, involving not more than 600 to 700 calories daily. But, for god's sake, do not try to count calories at each meal, because this is a sure way to failure. Calories must be translated into a menu before beginning your actual dieting. The diet should be comprised of normal food and not be a liquid or fad diet. One of the aims of this regime is to educate your appetite to be satisfied with low-calorie everyday foods.

Here is the general diet I usually give my patients. I have found it in the medical literature and modified it. It contains two meals, one in the morning and one in the late afternoon or evening.

Each meal should include the following foods:

(1) Four-ounce lean steak or 5 oz. of chicken (without fat and skin), or 6 oz. of lean saltwater fish, grilled or cooked without fat or oil.

(2) One large serving of raw or cooked vegetables, or a combination of vegetables, or a large helping of vegetable soup with no fat added. (Dried beans or other legumes, potatoes, rice, etc., are not vegetables.)

(3) One slice of bread, about half an inch thick.

(4) Half a lemon.

(5) One large apple or a medium-sized orange. You can wait and eat the fruit a few hours after the meal.

You can drink as much tea, coffee, or calorie-free soft drinks as you please during and between your two meals.

Salt, pepper, vinegar, sugar substitutes and other condiments are not limited.

No food is permitted between meals, except for the fruit mentioned above, and there is no dividing a meal into two parts.

This diet contains carbohydrates, proteins, even a little fat (in the meat and fish) and more than enough vitamins.

Meals can be taken whenever it is convenient and do not have to be eaten at the same hour every day. However, if you are working away from home, the first meal should be eaten before going to work and the second whenever you please after 5 p.m.

According to my experience this is an effective diet, but many others will do just as well, provided they conform to the principles outlined at the beginning of this chapter. If you find it easier to lose wight on some other diet—go right ahead.

If after you have been two or three weeks on a weight-losing diet, you are feeling down and terribly hungry, do not decide that you can add a little something here or there to your meals. This will not help you and you will feel terrible about this afterwards. It is a much better idea to go to a good restaurant, eat a regular meal, and the next morning you should continue your diet as before. If for any unforeseeable reason you find that you have to discontinue your diet for a while, not everything is lost. After the temporary interruption as described above (at which time you do not necessarily have to gorge yourself), you should go right back on your diet, until the fifteen-pound mark is finally reached.

How to Avoid
Regaining Lost Weight

The maintenance diet involves limiting the quantity of your food intake. You may, and should, eat almost everything except, of course, the very high calorie foods like cream, heavy desserts, chocolate, etc. You should eat with your family, at least for the main meal of the day. You should be sure to eat less than they do, and don't take large helpings of everything that is served on the table. Seconds are out!

The meals you eat alone should be kept small and low calorie—low-fat milk and cheese, many vegetables and fruits. Use Teflon-coated pans for frying with just a few drops of oil to prevent sticking. Have two to four meals a day, but take nothing in between.

When invited for coffee, do not tell the hostess that you are watching your weight. Chances are that she will start arguing with you. Let her put the cake on your plate, but don't eat it. Just nibble at it; be sure to leave most of it. When you go out to dinner with friends you do not have to eat the soup or other extraneous items that are served. Of the main dish you should eat as much as you think is good for you and leave the rest on the plate. On special occasions, when the food is very good, eat! One cannot and should not deprive oneself forever of good food. Just have small portions! And next day take only tea or coffee till dinner, to compensate for your good time the day before.

How do you know if you're eating too much? That is easy — your scales will clearly tell you. Weigh yourself every morning after going to the bathroom before getting dressed. I mean every morning! When you start to "forget" to weigh yourself, it is a sure sign that you are about to give in to food temptation. If you start gaining weight, cut down on your food consumption. If despite all precautions you have regained weight that you have lost, don't wait to amass ten or twenty pounds. After five pounds go back on the reducing diet for another ten days and afterwards continue the maintenance diet as before.

This advice is easy to give, but not easy to follow. Unfortunately there is no other way to keep your figure in shape. Many people are unable to diet consistently, not because they have a "weak character" or "no will power," but because it is extremely difficult to fight one's biological mechanisms.

Nevertheless, many do succeed. People who are in the limelight, like actors, models, socialites, politicians and their wives, will usually keep trim because their figure and public appearance is extremely important to them. We have seen that third generation American women are leaner than their mothers and grandmothers were at their age. It is a fact that women of the higher social classes weigh on the average less than those who are not well-off. So you can succeed. The price is high and one must always eat less than one wants, day in and day out. One must always be on guard to fight temptation. But this is the only way to achieve your weight-losing objective.

Don't be discouraged by the poor results reported by

medical studies, because these refer only to dieters who asked for medical help. These are the hard-core cases who did not succeed by themselves. Many do succeed in getting the upper hand over their appetite, and these are the people that do not appear in medical statistics.

Exercise

On the face of it, it would seem that one could eat more and simply get rid of extra calories by exercise. Theoretically this is true, but practically it almost never works. As we have seen before, appetite adjusts to the energy needs of the body and always aims to keep body weight constant. Exercise increases the appetite, sometimes a great deal and may make it difficult to adhere to a rigorous reducing diet. Moreover, it takes a lot of exercising to use up a substantial number of calories. It may take an hour of walking or half an hour of jogging to shed the amount of calories contained in one slice of bread with cheese. As far as the simple caloric count is concerned, not much will be lost.

While on a weight-loss diet it is not advisable to exercise more than you were used to prior to the diet. Low caloric diets are not hazardous to your health, but they may make you feel weak at times. So keep your exercise activities to levels you are used to.

As far as the simple calorie-equation is concerned, normal exercise will not do much for you, even when you are on a maintenance diet. However, there are other advantages to exercise. It will increase the elasticity of your muscles and skin, and it will help to retract the skin which hangs in folds around your arms and abdomen—if you are successful at losing weight. Some researchers believe that exercise performed regularly over a prolonged period of time can change the ratio between muscles and fat tissue in the body. Appetite may thus be balanced or adjusted at a somewhat lower level by the body itself. Unless you spend hours each day exercising, it is questionable whether exercise will measurably decrease your fat tissue, but it certainly is good for your figure, appearance, and well-being. Since maintenance diets are supposed to last for many years and become a way of life, sports and exercise should become part of it.

Children and Dieting

While Western society leans toward negative views about obesity, adults usually behave tactfully towards obese people. This is not so when it pertains to children's behavior to overweight children. They call their fat schoolmates names, and usually treat them cruelly. Parents of fat children, worried about their children's suffering and anxious about their health, are very eager to have them shed the excess weight. Unfortunately, this undertaking is doomed to failure, unless the child cooperates willingly. There is no way to make a child diet. Most adults do not succeed at dieting, so how can we expect children to do so? If parents try to restrict their children's food intake at home, it may only cause friction and frustration, unless the child truly wants to work at losing the extra weight. If kids are not committed to taking off the additional pounds, they will outsmart their parents by eating at friends' houses, buying food and finding many other ways to compensate for the calories they are deprived of at home.

Sometimes between the ages of thirteen to sixteen many girls become conscious of their figures and start to diet seriously. Usually, they don't consult parents or physicians but embark on a severe diet on their own. Many of these girls do manage to reduce until they find their figure satisfactory. Many of them go afterwards on a maintenance diet — without knowing the term — and manage to keep their weight down for many years, often until pregnancy and beyond. With boys it is more problematic, perhaps because they care less about their appearance. Some do succeed in losing weight by prolonged and vigorous exercise during their high school and college years.

Operations to Lose Weight

It is the dream of many a fat person, fighting food craving over the years, to have an operation which will end, once and for all, their obesity and their ordeal. Such a "dream operation" just does not exist.

There are two types of surgery for obesity. In one of them the small intestine is shortened. In the other, the upper part of the stomach is made into a very small pouch.

The small intestine operation attempts to prevent food absorption. Normally, all food is absorbed from the small intestine. Being about 18 feet long, it has a very large absorption surface. The operation leaves the upper twenty or so inches of the small intestine in place and connects the shortened part directly to the colon. All the rest of the small intestine is blocked, so that food no longer passes through. Fortunately, it is not cut away, but closed at both ends and left in the abdominal cavity. After this operation obese people lose a huge amount of fat, and their weight usually stabilizes at about ten to twenty percent above normal. Virtually all patients undergoing this operation were 100 percent overweight or more prior to the operation!

Weight loss does not depend on the patients' cooperation, since their bodies simply cannot absorb most of what they eat. The price they pay for this adjustment, however, is malabsorption, causing chronic diarrhea, which can be often very troublesome. As experience has accumulated, it has also become apparent that many essential substances were not being absorbed by the patient's shortened small bowel. Gallstones, kidney stones, a rheumatoid arthritis-like disease, electrolyte imbalance, and other diseases have also been frequently encountered as a result of the operation. In many patients the operation had to be reversed, i.e. the reconnecting of the section of the small bowel that was shut off. Today this operation has been virtually abandoned.

In the stomach operation, the stomach is divided into two unequal parts. The uppermost part of the stomach is made into a very small pouch, the volume of which is about one ounce. The pouch is surgically closed off from the rest of the stomach, with only a very small opening between the two parts. The patient cannot eat at a time more than minuscule quantities of solid food, because the upper part of the stomach—the pouch—can hold only one ounce. Liquid passes easily through the small opening between the pouch and the rest of the stomach. Weight loss is massive and proceeds till it stabilizes at about ten percent to twenty percent above normal. However, *losing this weight and keeping it off, depends on the patient's cooperation.* Some actually regain their weight by eating small quantities of fattening foods such as chocolate or other high-calorie food every few minutes. Others may drink large amounts of sweetened milk or cocoa, which are not arrested in the pouch, because liquid can pass freely through the small opening between the pouch and the other — large — part of the stomach.

Obese people are no gourmets. They eat to satisfy their appetite, preset at the level of their previous weight, which was about 100 percent above normal. It is no wonder that in some obesity recurs despite this operation. Moreover, their battle against appetite continues, though it is now greatly aided by their physical inability to down the large quantities of food they were used to consuming. Thousands of these stomach-shortening operations have been performed, but their merit is still not easy to evaluate. Long-range results are lacking and the operational procedure is still being adjusted. At present the operation is only advisable for people who are around 100 percent overweight. Among them, it is recommended only for those who feel that they are able to cooperate with their reduced stomach and will not try to overcome it with constant eating.

CHAPTER NINE

Climate and Your Health

Macro and Micro Climate

Mark Twain's famous statement that everybody talks about the weather but nobody does anything about it is no longer true. In his time almost all one could do was provide heat in apartments in the winter. Today the urban population in the affluent society lives almost year round in an artificial microclimate of comfort. Houses, public buildings, offices, work places, cars, and shops are all air-conditioned. A steadily increasing segment of the population seldom has to be exposed to the *natural* weather. From their air-conditioned homes in their air-conditioned cars, to their air-conditioned working places and from there to airconditioned shops, movie theaters, etc., and then back home.

Contrary to what was thought some time ago, life in an artificial microclimate is not hazardous to health. Going in and out of the microclimate into the natural air does not cause us any harm. It does not matter whether we leave a room heated to 75° (Fahrenheit) to go out into the freezing snow, or if we exit a cool room into humid heat in the nineties (Fahrenheit), provided, of course, that we are suitably dressed. One does not catch cold by briskly changing from heat to cold or vice versa— even many times daily.

In spite of all this, there is much to be said on how to live in comfort and in harmony with the weather. This, is beyond the scope of this book. I will however, make a few important points, directly affecting our health.

Tanning

The visible spectrum of the sun's rays spans from red to violet. Beyond this spectrum there are on the one end infrared rays, which provide mainly heat, and at the other end the ultraviolet rays. These ultraviolet rays, in high concentration, can cause damage to living cells and may even destroy them.

The human body has a defense mechanism that prevents ultraviolet light from penetrating deeper than the skin. The skin is composed of several layers of cells, which are easily penetrated by ultraviolet rays. Within the skin there are cells called melanocytes, which produce and disperse a black pigment around them called *melanin*. This pigment determines the color of our skin, eyes, and hair. Black-haired people have a great deal of melanin in their hair; they usually have dark eyes, due to the melanin in the iris of their eyes, and their skin is usually relatively dark for the same reason. Blonds have less pigment in their hair, they are often blue-eyed because there is little melanin in their iris, and they usually have a light complexion. The melanin of red-haired people is chemically somewhat different, and is responsible for the color of their hair and skin. The difference that melanin makes to our appearance and health can best be observed in albinos. They suffer from a genetically determined anomaly found in those having no melanin at all. This causes their hair to be completely white and their skin to be reddish. Sometimes, due to the absence of pigment from the iris, the blood vessels below their iris are visible, giving the eyes an unusual red color. This causes albinos great difficulties when looking at bright light. Negroes are black because they have more pigment in their skin, though the number of melanocytes in their skin is not greater than in Whites. Basically, the amount of melanin produced in all types of people is genetically determined.

Production of melanin in Whites is greatly influenced by exposure to ultraviolet light. It is a good example of a biological feedback mechanism. The more ultraviolet radiation and the greater the danger to the body's cells, the larger the protective melanin production. When exposed to ultraviolet light, white people's skin gets progressively darker, and in this way provides progressively greater protection from the sun's rays. The result is tanning. When exposure ceases, usually in autumn and winter, the skin reverts to its natural lighter color.

In the 19th Century, rickets were widespread in Europe, mainly in the North. When this disease strikes, it disturbs the normal ossification of children's bones. The bones become characteristically deformed, giving a very unsightly appearance, often for life. Rickets are caused by a vitamin D deficiency. Vitamin D is found in foods containing fat, such as milk and butter. A relative lack of these foods in the poorer strata of the population was the cause of the high incidence of rickets.

There is, however, also another source of vitamin D, namely the sun's rays. Ultraviolet light acts on certain chemical substances in the body, inducing their transformation into vitamin D. Not only was food lacking in the narrow streets of the poor in those Northern countries, but also missing was the sun.

When the sun's influence became widely known, the sun was suddenly sought after instead of avoided. Women were putting their parasols away. Mankind began to strip and enjoy the sun. Since this coincided with changes in moral attitudes, the transformation of the grotesque swimming and sports costumes from the beginning of this century into today's bikinis and sports briefs was quick in coming. Tanned skin became "in" and replaced the creamy complexion of the "girls with umbrellas." Today sporting a tan is a sign of health and prosperity, the trademark of the jet-set.

But it has also recently become apparent that sun-bathing is not an undivided blessing. Just as is the case in many other instances, what may be good and healthy in small quantities can become harmful in large doses. In other words, it is not true that when a little is good, more is even better. While this may be the case with money, it is certainly not the case with ultraviolet light. It is well known today that an excessive amount of ultraviolet light causes serious damage to the skin.

Solar radiation, especially ultraviolet radiation, is not evenly distributed throughout the globe. Because the axis of our planet is tilted toward the sun, the most exposed parts are the two so-called "desert belts" which encircle the earth around 300 North and again at 300 South. There is very little protective cloudiness in these desert belts, and radiation is strong and of long duration. Ultraviolet light is partially absorbed as it passes through the atmosphere; therefore it is strong on high mountains or on high elevations, where one tans very easily. On the other hand, at the Dead Sea, which is located 1200 feet below sea level, one has to be exposed for a relatively long period of time to tan. If the destruction of the protective ozone layer is not arrested, the quantity of ultraviolet light reaching the earth is going to increase significantly.

The nomadic inhabitants of North African and Asian deserts seem to know all about the harmful effect of excess radiation, as their bodies are always completely covered by garments reaching their ankles and sleeves that cover their wrists. Biologists, physicians, and other researchers have always wondered why these desert natives are completely covered by their garments despite the intense heat. They certainly act quite differently from what Europeans would do under the same circumstances, namely run around in shorts and sleeveless shirts. Many theories about the inhabitants' ways of dressing were put forward. Only now is it understood that these long garments effectively protect the skin from radiation.

Excessive ultraviolet radiation damages the skin. It first

causes thickening of the skin, giving it a leathery look. Premature ageing and wrinkling of the skin then follows. Later, discolorations and ulcers appear, mainly in red-haired people and those with light complexions. This is termed by dermatologists "farmer's skin" or "seamen's skin." Skin cancer is another likely occurrence. In countries with much radiation, the incidence of skin cancer is significantly higher than in Northern or Southern countries. This is well documented in Australia where immigrants from Britain with light complexions have a considerably higher incidence of skin cancer than their kin back home.

The danger of too much must be recognized and protective measures undertaken. There is no cause for panic, nor should we overact and avoid the sun completely. It is, as in many other instances, a quantitative problem and avoiding excess is sufficient.

Those who work outdoors and do not have the benefit of shade must learn to dress properly. Long pants, long sleeved shirts, and a broad-brimmed hat should be worn. In summer, when radiation is very strong, light-colored backgrounds, like sand, reflect the sun's rays, causing much additional indirect radiation. In these instances it is especially a good idea for those with light complexions to cover their faces with a protective lotion to block the sun.

For people on a sea or lake side vacation who want to tan, the following rules apply:

Do not sunbathe around noon, when radiation is strongest. It is best to take the sun in the morning before ten or ten thirty a.m. and in the afternoon after three o'clock.

Start out with ten minutes of exposure to the sun on the first day and add a few minutes every consecutive day, reaching a maximum of 30 minutes at a time.

Tanning lotions which contain PABA (para-amino-benzoic acid) undergo a chemical reaction when applied to the skin, which decreases the penetration of ultraviolet radiation. It takes about ten to fifteen minutes to create this reaction, so the lotion should be applied some time before going out into the sun. Your exposure time can be prolonged if protective lotions are used.

If you want to stay longer on the beach, put on a shirt and a hat that casts a shadow on your face. If you intend to spend several hours on a beach where there is no shade, it is advisable to bring along a beach umbrella or an open tent, or to tie a sheet to four poles. After and between sun-bathing and swimming, lie in the shadow. Even while in the shade you will still get some tan from the indirect radiation, reflected by the sand.

Careful with Snow-Shoveling

Surveys have shown that heart attacks are more frequent in winter than in summer. In the Northern hemisphere the peak time is usually in January. The reason is not known. One possibility is that the cold causes coronary arteries to contract, and this may compound the problems in arteries already damaged by arteriosclerosis. In the last few years, several papers have appeared in the medical literature reporting cases of heart attacks which occurred during snow-shoveling.

This may be because people went out into the cold insufficiently dressed, thinking: "I am just going out for a few minutes to clear out the driveway." Or they may not have been used to strenuous physical work. Snow shoveling is hard work, though one does not feel it at first. The last time they exerted themselves that heavily may have been a long time ago.

Again, there is no reason to panic. This happens to a very few of the millions who shovel snow every winter. But some precautions should be taken. If you are no longer young and not used to physical labor, leave the job to others. If you must do it, dress properly for the cold, use a small shovel to keep the weight of the snow down, and go about it slowly. Take a rest every few minutes. It is better to be late to work than to end up in the intensive care unit of your local hospital.

Alcohol and Cold Temperature

When outside temperature is high, the blood vessels in and under the skin widen greatly, producing what is termed physiologically vasodilatation. Our skin becomes flushed and hot. This helps us to dissipate excess body heat by radiating it to the surroundings. The reverse occurs in the cold. The blood vessels in the skin and in the tissues below the skin contract (vasoconstriction). Our skin feels cold and is pale or bluish. Heat loss to the surrounding is greatly decreased and the body's heat is preserved.

Alcohol has a paralyzing effect on the reactivity of small blood vessels to outside temperature, producing a devastating effect on the heat balance of our body. In hot climates it disturbs heat dissipation and predisposes to heatstroke. In the cold, vasoconstriction is delayed or does not occur at all. As a consequence, the body is losing a great amount of heat. Many cases are on record of drunk people who on the way home on a cold night had parts of their hands or feet frozen or in extreme cases have been found next morning completely frozen.

The obvious conclusion is that before or on exposure to a very hot or very cold environment one should steer clear of alcohol. But . . . everybody has heard or read about people out in the snow feeling cold and depressed until one of them passed around a bottle of liquor. Everybody took a hearty gulp and suddenly they felt warm and elated. What happened was that the alcohol counteracted the vasoconstriction. Warm blood flowed into the skin, producing a feeling of warmth and comfort. But, the body's defense mechanism against the cold has been pierced. People are losing heat and may pay a high price for the temporary feeling of well-being.

It is preferable to delay taking a shot of brandy or whiskey until arriving at a heated room—where vasodilation causes no harm and may even accelerate absorption of the surrounding heat into the blood stream.

Sauna?
No, Thank You!

For a very long time the sauna was popular mainly in Finland. During the sixties and seventies it became fashionable and suddenly spread to many countries. In 1976, at an international medical convention, a paper was presented by a Finnish doctor reporting a survey on the effects of the sauna. It turned out that during the year of the study, 89 people in Finland died in the sauna or immediately after leaving it!

Studies carried out in several other countries revealed additional evidence of the harmful effects of the sauna. People sweat profusely, sometimes losing one quart of water or more within twenty minutes. The heat and the sweating strain the heart, causing a very rapid heart rate and sometimes disturbances in its natural rhythm. Body temperature rises. All this may overload a clinically or latently diseased heart. Fainting and several types of cardiovascular accidents, sometimes resulting in death, have occurred as a result of just sitting in the sauna.

The possible beneficial effects of the sauna was the subject of several studies. No medical benefits were found. It does not prevent diseases and does not promote better functioning of any of the body's physiological mechanisms. The story that it cleans the pores of the sweat glands, or excretes "bad" substances from the blood is pure nonsense. The sweat glands are not dirty and do not need cleaning. The kidney is in charge of excreting unnecessary substances from the body and manages the job quite well.

If the sauna has no beneficial medical effects and on the other hand has already demonstrated that it may cause serious harm, why do so many people "feel so good" after spending time in a sauna? In the course of my own scientific investigations on the body's reactions to heat, I have kept paid volunteers in climatic chambers at temperatures and humidity levels equivalent to those of the sauna. The subjects of the experiment were never told anything about sauna. They were told that effects of heat on the body were being investigated. After a short while they started to complain about feeling weak and that the heat or humidity or both were uncomfortable and intolerable. This serves to prove how our reactions and feelings are often influenced by the power of suggestion. The sauna is a classic example. Since people have been influenced over the years to believe that a sauna is "good for you," and that they are supposed to come out feeling refreshed and in a better state of health—just like all those healthy Swedish and Danish people—they start believing that they also feel better after taking saunas.

There is actually no good reason to recommend the use of a sauna. The recommendation should be not to use it. But if you like saunas, despite all that is known about them make sure of the following:

- Exposure time should not exceed ten minutes for people below forty-five years and five minutes for people above forty-five.

- People with heart disease or high blood pressure should avoid their use altogether.

- Cold drinks should be available in the immediate vicinity of the sauna.

- A rest period of at least thirty minutes before entering the sauna is imperative. Never enter a sauna immediately following physical exertion like a tennis game or weight lifting.

How Much to Drink in Summer

During the summer months we must drink more because in addition to the usual fluid requirements of the body, we must replace water that is lost through perspiration. Thirst is not a good enough indicator of the body's fluid requirements. As long as people are in their habitual surroundings, they rely on their past consumption levels and experience as to how much they need to drink to maintain their body's water balance. But when they go on vacation, for instance, traveling in warmer climates, participating in walking tours, or lying for hours on the beach, they may unknowingly become dehydrated. The question of how to avoid dehydration under such circumstances arises.

The amount of sweat excreted daily depends on many factors; the temperature, the humidity, hours of exposure to the heat, degree of physical exertion and type of clothing worn, among others. It may vary from about two quarts a day in an air-conditioned room and doing little physical work to twelve quarts or more, when engaged in strenuous labor on a hot day. Since conditions change, not only from day to day but sometimes from one minute to another, it is futile to try to calculate how much a person perspires on any given day.

The only realistic way to tell if you are becoming dehydrated is to look at the color of the urine. The kidney's job is to keep constant the body fluids. As soon as even slight dehydration occurs, the kidneys increase water reabsorption from the urine fluid. Urine quantity decreases and consequently becomes more concentrated (or darker in color).

The normal 24-hour quantity of urine for the average person who is not dehydrated is about a quart and a half. Obviously no one is going to measure daily urine output! But this really isn't necessary. The more concentrated the urine, the darker its color. You are generally not dehydrated if you have very light-colored urine with a watery or straw-colored hue. Darker urine indicates incipient dehydration, and you should recognize from this that it is time to drink.

What to Drink?

It really makes no difference what beverage is used to replace the water lost in sweat and urine, as long as we drink enough. When the need arises to drink a lot, as when working or walking in the heat, cold drinks are preferable because they are downed quickly and they have also a cooling effect on the body. It makes no difference whether we drink water, soda, tea, coffee, or other beverages.

Sometimes the question arises whether tap water is fit to drink. Almost everywhere and at all times tap water poses no problem. However, in some areas tap water is unsafe to drink due to the presence of larger than normal amounts of chemical or biological contaminants. There are standards of permissibility for public water supplies. They are regularly tested and if contaminated, the public is usually alerted. In such cases boiling the tap-water is usually sufficient to make it safe.

If tap water is unpalatable, due to chlorination or other reasons, to a degree that one is ready to spend money on buying water, there is a large choice: Mineral water has a higher mineral content than tap-water; Seltzer and club soda are filtered and artificially carbonated tap water; spring and well water are usually agreeable to the palate. However, bottled water is not always sufficiently tested, as the Perrier recall has shown. If one buys regularly from one company, it is advisable to inquire whether their product is tested periodically.

And let us not forget that many vegetables and fruits have a high water content. Table 8 demonstrates that some of them contain 80 percent and even 90 percent water. They are a source of fluid for those who don't feel like drinking much liquid.

TABLE 8
WATER CONTENT (PERCENTAGES) OF
VEGETABLES AND FRUITS

Banana	73%
Avocado	75
Potato, cooked	78
Grapes	82
Pear	83
Apple	84
Peach	86
Grapefruit	89
Cabbage	91
Tomato	93
Melon	93
Watermelon	93

CHAPTER TEN

Keeping Away from Cancer's Claws

What Is Cancer?

Our body is composed of many billions of cells of different types and functions. These cells, each with a nucleus in its center, form tissues and organs. The life span of the cells varies. In some types of cells it is measured in days, in others in months and years. Dead cells are replaced by new ones, produced according to the body's needs.

Cancer is an inordinate and uncontrolled growth of cells, which reproduce unrelated to the body's needs. They may reproduce in a certain area, giving rise to a tumor which invades the surrounding tissues, or they may travel with the blood stream to distant parts of the body producing daughter colonies named metastases.

Cancer is not a new disease. It has been known for thousands of years, and "chemotherapy" in the form of arsenic was applied some 2500 years ago. But not much is known about the incidence of cancer in the past. The apparent increase in modern times is mainly due to the prolongation of life, since cancer occurs mostly in middle and old age. And it is not one disease but a group of diseases, related in character; each type in each organ is due to different causes.

What Causes Cancer?

In spite of many years of epidemiological, clinical, and experimental research, our knowledge is still fragmentary. The processes which induce billions of cells in our body to grow and reproduce in an orderly way are extremely complicated. Sometimes one wonders why more cells do not behave imperfectly when they divide and grow. Perhaps some do, and are inhibited or destroyed by the proper body's immune system. But practically speaking it is important for the reader to know which influences foreign to our body play a role in the causation of cancer tumors.

Smoking

It is absolutely beyond doubt that cigarette smoking causes cancer of the lung. Epidemiology (the branch of medicine dealing with the incidence and distribution of disease) proves it clearly. The incidence of cancer correlates with the patterns of cigarette smoking; the more one smokes, the higher the risk. In heavy smokers the risk of lung cancer is ten times that of nonsmokers. In the six decades in which most smokers switched from other forms of smoking to cigarettes, the incidence of lung cancer in men increased twenty-five times! Lung cancer was almost unknown in women when women hardly smoked at all. Since they started to emulate men, they too show a very steep increase in the incidence of lung cancer. It is astounding that switching from other uses of tobacco, like chewing, pipe and cigar smoking to cigarettes, has had such a profound and terrible effect (for further details see pages 100–101).

Alcohol

Cancer of the liver is common in Southeast Asian countries and is ascribed to the ingestion of various toxic materials. It is rare in Europe and North America, except in people who suffer from cirrhosis, a severe liver disease caused by alcohol abuse (for further details see page 91).

Occupational Hazards

In some occupations people come into contact with carcinogenic, or cancer-causing, substances. The first and most famous instance was reported in London 200 years ago. Many cases of cancer of the scrotum, normally an extremely rare occurrence, were reported in London chimney sweepers. It was found that the soot penetrated their clothing and accumulated in the wrinkles around the scrotum. Repeated irritation finally produced cancer. Another more recent example is workers in the aniline dye industry who showed an unusually high incidence of bladder cancer. The chemical aniline, used to produce dye, entered the body in small quantities during their work and was concentrated in the kidney and excreted in the urine. On its way out of the body aniline-laden urine stayed for some time in the bladder, causing irritation of its lining and finally producing cancer.

Solar Radiation

Other tumors clearly associated with external influences are tumors of the skin. It is definitely established that ultraviolet radiation irritates the skin, especially of people with light complexion. During repeated and prolonged exposure, among other damage, it causes a high incidence of skin cancer (for further detail see pages 130–34).

Decreasing Incidence of Some Cancers

Cancer of the uterine cervix was the most common form of cancer in women forty years ago. Its incidence was related to the early onset of sexual intercourse, promiscuity, and poor hygiene. Its disproportionately low incidence among Jewish women led to the conclusion that in uncircumcised males a carcinogenic substance is found under the foreskin. The incidence of this type of cancer is now about one third what it used to be. This decrease is attributed mainly to better hygiene and to the widespread custom of circumcision.

Not all cancers can be attributed to known predisposing external factors. The incidence of gastric cancer, for instance, varies greatly in different parts of the world. Though its incidence is now decreasing everywhere, it is still much higher in Japan and in Iceland than in the West. Some researchers blame the high incidence in Japan on the consumption of raw or smoked fish, but this has not been definitely proven, nor is it known why the incidence in the U.S is now about one fourth of what it once was.

Other types of cancer also differ in incidence geographically. Cancers of the colon and rectum and of the prostate in men and breast and ovaries in women are much more common in Europe and North America than in underdeveloped countries. The reasons have not yet been elucidated. However, differences in incidence related to geographical and social factors leave no doubt that environmental influences are involved. Japanese, Blacks and Asians, who live in the U.S.A. acquire the incidence pattern of the U.S.A., instead of those of their native country.

Fiber and Roughage

Cancer of the colon and rectum is being linked to constipation and the long time that food remains in the gastrointestinal tract. Studies showed that the average time between ingestion of food and excretion of its remnants is ten to fourteen hours in Blacks living in traditional African villages as compared to twenty four to thirty eight hours in urban Whites. It must be pointed out, however, that the connection between cancer of the colon and rectum and the length of time food remains in the gut, though very plausible, has not yet been definitely proven. Nevertheless, doctors today advise patients to eat more fiber, in order to hasten the passage of food. (See pages 71–72.)

Internal Factors?

Studies show approximately that one out of twenty people smoking two packs of cigarettes daily for thirty years, and one out of five who smoke three packs daily for forty years, will develop lung cancer. This shows that environmental factors, important as they may be, are not the only ones operating. Internal factors play an important role as well. The susceptibility of the tissue (in this case the lung), its reaction to the irritant, the strength of the immune system, availability of neutralizing substances, and other unknown or partially known factors, some of them genetic, are what is truly decisive. Furthermore, even nonsmokers do sometimes get lung cancer, though this is very rare.

At the present stage of our knowledge there is little we can do about the internal factors. We must concentrate on the elimination of the recognized external carcinogenic substances. On the face of it, this is a logical and obvious thing to do. But in practice it can be rather complicated because not always are the damaging substances known and in other instances it is very difficult to eliminate the incriminated substances.

"Zero-Hypothesis" and the Definition of Poison

The "Zero-Hypothesis" postulates that we must completely avoid even the smallest quantities of carcinogenic substances. The so-called "Delaney Clause" is based on this theory. It was introduced in 1958 as a supplement to the law governing the FDA (Food and Drug Administration). According to this clause, no substance can be sold as food or as a drug or be used in food production if it has been shown to have a carcinogenic effect on human or animals, regardless of dosage.

Besides the fact that it is practically impossible to adhere to this clause, as we shall see later, its theoretical basis is scientifically untenable. "Carcinogens" have toxic or poisonous effects. Let us examine the definition of poison. Poison is a substance causing harm to our body or parts thereof, in very small quantities. In other words, there is no way to define poison without linking it to a certain dosage. For example, carbon monoxide, a tasteless and colorless gas, is present in the air at a concentration of up to ten parts per million. It causes no harm whatsoever and we live with it all our lives. However, a concentration of 800 parts per million causes poisoning and death within hours. Many drugs used in medicine have a lifesaving effect in their proper dosage, but are harmful and even fatal if the dosage is increased. This is also true not only for external substances but also for substances produced within the body. Hormones, which at physiological levels regulate many metabolic process essential to health, may cause severe diseases if produced in excess. On the other hand, many toxic substances are practically harmless if sufficiently diluted.

On this basis alone the zero-hypothesis must be considered overzealous and unscientific. An analogous approach would be to say "Let us eliminate the thyroid gland, because its hormones, if produced in excess, cause thyrotoxicosis." *Quantitating risk is essential to all our activities in life*; eating or drinking, sleeping or working, exercising or resting, each is essential in the right quantity. Too little or too much of anything may be harmful and even dangerous.

Sugar Substitutes

A good example is artificial sweeteners like cyclamate and saccharine. When cyclamate was fed to rats in enormous quantities, corresponding to 3000 tablets a day in humans, some of the rats developed tumors of the bladder. The use of cyclamate was quickly forbidden in the United States, in accordance with Delaney's clause.

The zero-hypothesis argument is this: We can assume that 3000 tablets a day will cause tumors in the bladder of a certain percentage of users. How can we be sure that users of thirty tablets (one hundredth of the dose!) will not get a tumor in one out of a million or out of ten million? This undoubtedly is true. But it is just as true that one or more out of a million will get a tumor in the bladder without ever having been exposed to even one tablet of cyclamate, just as there are people who get lung cancer without ever having smoked cigarettes. On the other hand, cyclamate is very useful for diabetics, who cannot use sugar, and for people fighting obesity, which is harmful in itself. Cyclamate could substitute for twenty teaspoons of sugar, or about 400 calories daily, without causing the slightest damage. Many studies performed on healthy and sick people using cyclamate, failed to produce any evidence of harmful effects. Instead of prohibiting the production and sale of cyclamate, the public should have been told to restrict its intake to no more than thirty of forty tablets daily which is more than anyone would ever want to use anyway. This in fact has been done in several countries.

The banning of cyclamate was not only unnecessary, but even harmful. It would most probably never have passed in Congress were it not for pressure from the sugar lobby and other interest groups. Incidentally, it should be mentioned that public nutrition is not guided by scientific principles. Food growing, producing, and marketing is a substantial part of the economy, and special interest groups have a great influence on what we eat or do not eat. Had the public not protested violently, saccharin would also have been banned, as it actually should be in accordance with Delaney's clause.

Beyond these theoretical considerations, it is virtually impossible to eat anything even remotely resembling a normal diet if one adhered to this zero-hypothesis. Even "natural" food will not do. Carcinogenic substances have been found in many plants and other items which are an essential part of our daily diets. A paper summarizing our knowledge about dietary carcinogens and anticarcinogens was published in 1983, in the prestigious scientific journal *Science*. It begins by stating that ". . . plants in nature synthesize toxic chemicals in large amounts, apparently as a defense against the hordes of bacterial, fungal, insect, and other animal predators." The paper goes on to describe sixteen carcinogenic substances found in plants. These carcinogens are: safrole in many edible plants and in black pepper; hydrazine in edible mushrooms;

furocoumarins in celery, parsnips, figs, parsley, and citrus oil; solanine in potatoes. Flavonoids and quinones are extremely widespread, about one gram is contained in the daily human diet. Theobromine in cocoa powder, chocolate, tea. Pyrrolizidine is present in thousands of plant species, herbs, herbal teas, and honey. Gossypol is present in cottonseed and its crude oil. Sterculic acid is widespread in oils from various seeds and in fish, poultry, eggs, and milk from animals fed on cottonseed. Alfalfa sprouts contain a highly toxic substance. Nitrite and derivates are found in beets, celery, lettuce, spinach, radishes, and rhubarb. Even burnt and browned material, like bread crust, toast, steak, and coffee, are also carcinogenic. The paper concludes that ". . . the human dietary intake of natural pesticides is likely to be several grams a day—probably 10,000 times higher than the dietary intake of man-made pesticides"!

This is a partial list, but it shows that going through life without eating carcinogenic substances is just impossible. Protecting ourselves from cancer by trying to eliminate all traces of any carcinogenic substance is like trying to rid the planet of infectious disease by attempting to completely avoid any contact with bacilli and viruses. This would be futile and doomed to failure from the onset, and also unnecessary. Our body has ways and means to cope with many bacilli, even virulent ones. And contact with bacilli strengthens our defense mechanism against infection.

The same goes for carcinogenic substances. In our food, sometimes in the same items that contain the carcinogens, there are also anticarcinogens. Another human line of defense is the periodic shedding of the cells lining the skin and the gastrointestinal tract. We also have our immune mechanism and other means to destroy dangerous or damaged cells. It is logical to believe that if the human body didn't have these powerful built-in mechanisms how could any of us have survived beyond our early childhood?

The fact is that carcinogens are widespread in nature. We may ingest several grams daily, even 10,000 times more than the content of chemical pesticides in our food. And what a clamor was raised in the press about the danger of pesticides, although many of them were tested and retested and shown not to be carcinogenic to humans? This only proves that the people supposedly protecting society sometimes act without understanding or checking on the facts. How many people are spending good money to buy "organic" food and herbs to make sure that they do not ingest any carcinogenic substances. And look how they "feel better" and so much "healthier" than the poor fools still "poisoning themselves" with normal diets.

The Cancer Scare

As if people were not frightened enough of everything related to cancer, the press and media have made the cancer scare one of their favorite preoccupations. Every other day a new substance is reported to be "carcinogenic." One day it is coffee, the next it is smoked meat or fish, boiled food, even the crust of bread, or cooking oil that is reused. Someone has found carcinogens in almost every kind of food. We are even told that by cooking meat a carcinogenic substance is produced. The sequence of events usually goes as follows: A researcher presents a paper at a conference, relating findings of theoretical or methodological interest. A reporter, out to get a scoop, will make a sensation of it in the press or on T.V. In the process significance, scientific quantifications, and practical implications are lost. The scare is on. As the old proverb goes, "If a fool throws a stone into the water, even twenty wise men may not be able to retrieve it."

How should one react to this flood of "news"? If food eaten for generations, or prepared in conventional, time honored ways is implicated, you should take the new report with a grain of salt. After all, mankind has survived for so long eating the newly indicted foods—so maybe they cannot be all that bad. What really matters is the quantitative approach. If coal residues, which form on a grilled steak, are carcinogenic, let us not confine our diet to steaks three times daily, day in day out, and make it our exclusive food. Actually, the rule that should guide us all along applies here as well. One should eat a large variety of foods, prepared in different ways, with obvious seasonal variations. If we do this, we will get all the essential substances and not eat too much of any food which may be harmful in large quantities.

A somewhat more careful approach is required with regard to artificially prepared food and food additives. Here too we should practice moderation. In addition, naturally every new chemical substance used in food growing and processing should be thoroughly tested to detect the truly harmful ones.

Other Means of Prevention

Although many more people succumb to cardiovascular disease than to cancer, the latter seems to be more frightening. The reason may be the fear of the unknown, so common to man. Cancer is regarded as a fatal disease, the appearance of which cannot be foreseen or obviated and which is often tantamount to a death sentence.

These notions of cancer are inaccurate. Many cancers are preventable. All occupational cancers can be avoided by eliminating the causative substances or providing safe working conditions. Lung cancer can be almost completely eradicated by non-smoking. The incidence of skin cancer can be greatly reduced by avoiding excessive exposure to solar radiation. Cancers of the colon and rectum are, apparently, related to faulty eating habits, higher fiber content in the diet will most probably diminish their incidence. Cancer of the uterine cervix and of the stomach are already on the decrease, for reasons as yet not completely accounted for.

This list shows that, contrary to prevailing popular beliefs, much can be done. People are too often led by "naturalistic" gurus and by adherents of the zero-hypothesis to seek salvation in the wrong places. And—above all—cancer is treatable. With methods available today, including surgery, x-ray radiation, and chemotherapy, about half of the cancer patients now survive.

Checkup?

One of the major problems in the diagnosis and treatment of cancer is early detection. Obviously, the earlier and smaller the tumor is when treatment begins, the better the outlook. The trouble is that a small tumor usually produces no symptoms. At this stage people are not aware that anything is wrong, they feel no pain, and consequently do not seek treatment.

To promote early detection, preventive periodic examinations are suggested. Experience, however, has shown that with the present diagnostic methods, the results of these examinations are often unreliable. Statistics do not indicate a significantly better prognosis in cases that were detected in the course of periodic examination, than in those diagnosed after symptoms appeared. Even the famous "Pap" smear, used to detect cervical cancer, has not stood the test of time. The drastic decrease in incidence and mortality from cancers of the cervix has also been observed in countries where these tests were not made. Today, considerably less emphasis is put on the test and the suggested interval between smears has been considerably prolonged.

It is a good idea to be examined once yearly by your family physician. The doctor may detect newly developed hypertension, diabetes, heart disease, or even a tumor in the breast or skin. One should certainly go for medical examination as soon as any symptom appears, be it newly developed constipation or diarrhea, a persistent cough, blood in the urine, feces, or sputum, or any other deviation from the normal — do not delay, call your physician at once.

The best way to detect breast cancer very early is monthly self-examination. By inspection in front of a mirror and a thorough palpation, a woman will be able to detect even a slight change in the appearance or consistency of her breasts. Immediate medical attention to a small tumor significantly facilitates treatment and greatly increases the chances of success.

Stop the Nonsense!

In the foregoing chapters the reader has been warned several times not to act on the "most recent findings," as they are reported in the newspapers and media. Such warnings may be conceived as unscientific, and may appear to be in contrast to the state of mind of modern society—which assumes, *a priori,* that the new, and certainly the newest, is always an improvement over the old. There are, however, many good reasons why that is not so, as far as medical research is concerned. Some of these will be explained below.

The black dots in the accompanying figure represent holes found in an actual archeological dig. Some may be post holes, others rabbit holes, or whatever. One group of archeologists selects a set of holes as post holes and rejects others as irrelevant. They then join their "data" to come up with hypothetical early huts—the interrupted lines of the left-most drawing. When these "data" appear in print, they are the "most recent findings."

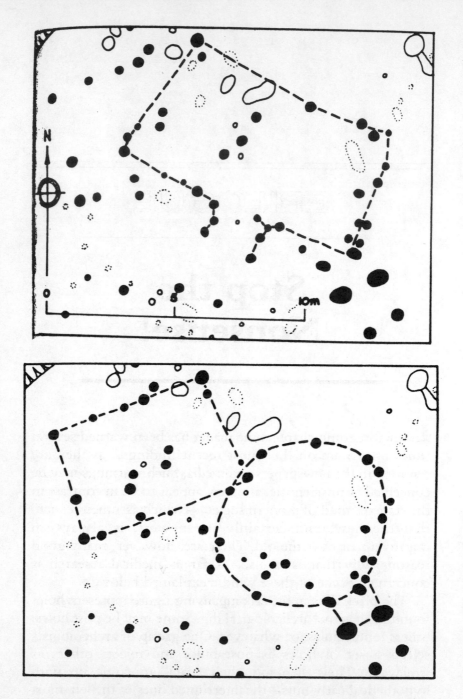

(From R.L. Gregory and E.H. Gambrich, eds., *Illusion in Nature and Art,* London: Gerald Duckworth & Co., 1973)

Then comes another group of archeologists, who select some *different* holes as "data" and come up with different hypothetical huts (the right-most drawing). *These,* then, are the "most recent findings."

What is the truth? Either of the two groups may eventually be proven to be right — or they may both be wrong! Further research, employing other methods and different disciplines — done perhaps by architects, carpenters, contractors, etc. — will bring to light more and more "data." It may take years until the true state of affairs is revealed, or until at least a reasonable hypothesis is reached.

Though they are illustrative of my point, archeological data do not have a direct bearing on our lives, however. Nevertheless, if the findings concerned nutrition, would we not be at a loss as to what to believe? If, today, we rush out to buy, for example, broccoli — believing it to be our salvation — and tomorrow the newspapers report that somebody has found, in a batch of broccoli, a substance thought to be carcinogenic, then broccoli will immediately be considered dangerous. If the newspaper item neglects to inform us that the quantity of the carcinogenic substance is minuscule, even negligible, and not different from that found in other vegetables, then broccoli will be considered by most people as a dangerous vegetable and will be avoided. Unfortunately, there is much "medical" reportage in the mass media today that is not as accurate and informed as it should be.

By such reportage, you have a right to feel confused and betrayed. In the days — not long past — when decaffeinated coffee was assaulted by the "most recent findings" (which were not confirmed, and were finally recanted), a newspaper story told about a man who changed from regular coffee to decaf, believing it to be more healthful, and who now felt betrayed. "First, it's good, then it's bad," he said. "I told my secretary, 'My decaf days are over. Bring me bottled water.' She said, 'Haven't you heard? Bottled water's bad now. No fluorides.'"

A company researching food marketing in New Jersey polled thousands of consumers and reported that upwards of 80 percent complained of "confusion and conflicting health information when it comes to food."

Very often, newspaper copy is presented in a way that obscures everything except the obvious practical implication. Here is an example: "Four years ago, a biochemist in Wisconsin began baking bread, cookies, etc., with flaxseed oil, which is rich in omega-3 fatty acids. A study by Dr. L.T., at the University of Toronto, found that in addition to its cholesterol-lowering ability, flaxseed oil caused a 50 percent reduction in pre-cancer cells in laboratory animals."

What are we expected to do after reading this piece of information? Here is a food item that will save you not only from heart attacks but also from cancer?! Out we rush to the supermarket to buy flaxseed oil and, if available, also bread baked with this great oil. . . . But wait a minute. Let's have a second look. Who *bakes bread with oil* or with more than a very small amount? Has the research proven that this brand of bread decreases blood cholesterol and pre-cancerous cells? And if so, by how much? What does the researcher mean by pre-cancerous cells? How often do these cells give rise to cancer? What animals were studied? How much flaxseed oil was used, and in what form, to achieve the reported results? Has the effect of other oils been checked and compared. . .?

After considering these and many other questions that come to mind, it appears that we can hang up our coat again, stay home, and go on eating our regular bread. The whole matter, in the way it was presented, sounds very much like a smart piece of commercial promotion.

Another thing to consider is that we never know who really has ordered the research that yields such surprise findings. Health is a big industry. Be it sport shoes, spas, vitamins and minerals—and especially food—big money is involved. Much is spent on direct and indirect advertising. In an avocado-producing country, growers inserted an ad in the newspapers calling for a researcher "to examine the theory that avocado increases sexual prowess." The ad itself was intended to increase sales. We do not know whether a researcher indeed applied, but who could design a scientific method to prove or disprove the "theory"? Attributing increased sexual prowess to food lies more in the realm of beliefs (and hopes); it is not easily verifiable through scientific "facts."

There is no way to halt the glut of information, and misinformation, disseminated about health. Every producer will continue to push his "health product"; newspapers and the media will continue to print "health news" that caters to the public's interest. And there is no easy way to quickly verify the efficacy of these products that, it is claimed, promote health and/or longevity. It may be years until the truth about them is discovered.

In the meantime. . .? Try to take the "health news" with a grain of salt. Do not act on the news hysterically, but wait until doctors reach some kind of consensus, and listen to your own doctor's advice or to what *reliable medical authorities* have to say. Don't be afraid to "miss the boat." You have, doubtless, lived many years without, say, avocado or oat bran. Another year or two won't do you any harm.

It is no wonder, of course, that the quest for more and newer information on health—even instant health—leads not only to our confusion but also undermines our trust in science. After several on/off experiences, say with decaffeinated coffee or oat bran, many people will say, "To hell with it! *Everything* they say may be wrong. I am going back to gravy and butter!" Or, as expressed by a *New York Times* columnist, "If cholesterol had not existed, it would have had to be invented. Now some people are saying maybe it was."

The hysterical interest today in health, and the compulsion to pick up on every fad, has something unhealthy, even morbid in it. More and more people have come to have a hypochondriacal outlook on life. How-to-improve-one's-health-instantly has become their main topic of conversation, and a good portion of their energy and time are devoted to this end. One of the consequences is a continuous guilt-feeling about any kind of digression or "health sin." Disease has become not only a horror but also a disgrace—something that one has brought onto oneself, something that could have been avoided.

Except for smoking—which is truly dangerous in any amount —forget about the fads, don't react hysterically to the latest promotional ads and "health news." Stick, instead, to a *healthful life-style that is in accordance with already-well-established* scientific fact. Such a life-style will not automatically assure you of greater longevity or greater immunity to disease, but it will make for a better quality of life and decrease your chances of acquiring serious disease, something that may cause you suffering or even death.

Besides eliminating smoking, it is also a good idea to curtail your intake of alcoholic beverages if you are a regular drinker. As for exercise, experience some of the kind that you like and *that is appropriate to your age,* leaving jogging to the very young, if you are not in that age group, and marathon races to the professionals. If you like coffee, drink it but do not abuse it; five cups a day should satisfy you — if, indeed, you need that much.

Try, too, to keep to a reasonable weight — not by trying a new diet every other week, but by maintaining the weight you have succeeded in reaching after a reasonable amount of deprivation.

About stress...One cannot run away from all one's troubles and sorrows: These are part of life. So do not bemoan the "terrible stress" you are under, blaming it for your health problem(s), if any. Taking life's problems in a more philosophical vein may be helpful to both your physical and mental health. Also, aim to keep your blood cholesterol below 220 milligrams. This will reduce your chances of suffering a heart attack. Though people with low blood cholesterol levels are, in fact, having heart attacks less often these days than those with high levels, the low-cholesterol people do not, on the average, live any longer. Especially for people with a family history of cardiac or vascular, and for those who have one or more additional risk factors (such as hypertension, diabetes, and obesity), lowering blood cholesterol is of course of great benefit.

Finally, as for your diet: Eat a varied one, composed of many items. Have an assortment of vegetables and fruit, which supply you with necessary vitamins, minerals, and fiber. Do not be too aggressive when using the salt shaker, of course. There is no reason for you to shun meat, but keep your intake of it low-fat, and substitute fish for it twice weekly. (Remember that the idea that meat is not a "natural" food has no basis in fact.) Use low-fat milk products; many of them are very tasty.

If you stick to the above suggestions, there is absolutely no need for health-store supplements such as vitamins or minerals — and certainly not fish-oil pills — many of which may have undesirable side effects.

How to *Stop the Nonsense!* has been outlined in the chapters of this book. Adhering to the advice given will permit you to lead a healthier, more normal life and avoid what is known today to affect you adversely.

To your health!